Anatomy of the Body

The Art of Human Physiology

N.P. James

Cv/Visual Arts Research Series 10

Cv /Visual Arts Research Series 10

ANATOMY OF THE BODY

The Art of Human Physiology

ISBN: 9781706212744

Cv/Visual Arts Research Series ISSN 1476-9980

Publication copyright © 2013 Cv Publications

The right of Nicholas Philip James to be identified as the author of this work has been asserted in accordance with sections 77 and 78 of the Copyright, Designs and Patents Act 1988

All rights reserved; no part of this publication may be stored in a retrieval system, or transmitted in any form or by any means, electronic, mechanical, photocopying, recording, or otherwise, without the prior written permission of the Publishers. Except in the United States of America, this book is sold subject to the condition that it shall not, by way of trade or otherwise be lent, re-sold, hired out, or otherwise circulated without the publisher's prior consent in any form of binding other than that in which it is published and without a similar condition including this condition being imposed on the subsequent publisher.

Anatomy of the Body
was first published in 2001 with a second edition in 2006.
The third revised and enlarged edition is published in April 2013

Cv Publications
www.tracksdirectory.ision.co.uk

Cv/Visual Arts Research

Formed in 1995 Cv/*Visual Arts Research* is a documentary resource of developments in contemporary art. The survey began in April 1988, and was first published as the quarterly review *Cv Journal of Art and Crafts*. *Cv* was produced until 1992 and the collection of interviews, features and reviews provided the foundation of the Cv/*VAR* archive and subsequent publications.

Following *Cv Journal* the data-base shifted towards digital process offering for greater flexibility of publication. Cv/*VAR* addresses the fields of academic research, galleries and museums worldwide, and a growing non-specialist readership. In this respect the archive has been organised as a file system which may be accessed as individual articles or collated volumes, according to specific requirements. The programme is categorized as *Interviews-Artists; Curators-Collections; Crafts Directory; Histories; Social Studies and Studio Work*. There are now over one hundred and fifty titles published in the series. Forty folios from Cv/Visual Arts Research archive were published through 2006, documenting projects and series realised between 1972 and 2006. Each title contains full colour prints of artwork with related documentation.

In Cv/VAR series no.10, *Anatomy of the Body,* 112 panel paintings made in 2001 and 2013 by N.P.James constructed a metaphor for the human physical system. A viscous surface of pulped and washed colour interprets the intricate framework of muscles, arteries, bone and soft tissue, all infused with an internal dynamic of potent nervous energy.

The volume carries colour reproductions of the artworks with descriptions of the location and function of portrayed parts.

Anatomy of the Body

Panel paintings made by Philip James ROI in 2001 and 2013 constructed a metaphor for the human physical system. A viscous surface of pulped and washed colour interprets the intricate framework of muscles, arteries, bone and soft tissue, all infused with an internal dynamic of potent nervous energy. First published as Cv/VAR series 10, 2001, the volume includes further studies made in 2013 with descriptions of the location and function of portrayed parts.

Contents

Anatomy 2001
Aorta 5
Arch of Atlas 5
Arm 6
Artery 6
Atrium 7
Bladder 7
Bones 8
Brain 8
Branches 9
Breast 9
Bronchi 10
Bulb 10
Buttocks 11
Canal 11
Capillary 12
Cartilage 12
Cavity 13
Cell 13
Cerebellum 14
Cervix 14
Column 15
Conchae 15
Cornea 16
Cuneiform 16
Diaphragm `7
Digits 17
Disks 18
Ducts 18
Duodenum 19
Ear 19
Esophagus 20
Fascia 20

Femur 21
Fibula 21
Finger 22
Fissure 22
Follicle 23
Foot 23
Gland 24
Gonadotropins 24
Heart 25
Heel 25
Hip 26
Intestine 25
Iris 27
Jaw 27
Knee 28
Knuckle 27
Labia 29
Labyrinth 29
Lung 30
Metatarsal 30
Mouth 31
Neck 31
Nucleus 32
Orifice 32
Pelvis 33
Perineum 33
Pigment 34
Pubis 34
Rectum 35
Retina 35
Rib Cage 36
Sacrum 35
Scalp 37

Shin 37
Shoulder 38
Skin 38
Skull 39
Spine 39
Spleen 30
Stomach 40
Teeth 41
Testicle 41
Thorax 42
Thumb 42
Throat 43
Tongue 43
Veins 44
Wrist 44

Anatomy 2013
Axons 46
Bile Duct 47
Bone Marrow 48
Deltoids 49
Diaphragm 50
Epidermis 51
Fibres 52
Filaments 53
Gallbladder 54
Humerus 55
Intestine 56
Ions 57
Kidney 58
Levers 59
Liver 60
Lymph Nodes 61

Meninges 62
Molecules 63
Monocytes 64
Motor 65
Mucus 66
Nails 67
Neurons 68
Nerves 69
Ovary 70
Pancreas 71
Phosphate 72
Plasma 73
Prostate 74
Receptors 75
Saliva 76
Semen 77
Synapse 78
Sesamoid 79
Spleen 80
Sternum 81
Taste Buds 82
Testes 83
Tubules 84
Urethra 85
Uterus 86
Vertebrae 87
Womb 88

Disclaimer: The information presented on this publication is strictly for educational purposes only. It by no means constitutes a recommendation of treatment or substitute for medical consultations. Medical knowledge is dynamic. Whilst every care has been taken to ensure the accuracy and up-to-date-ness of the content of this publication, Cv Publications or its owners or partners will not accept responsibility or liability of any sort for the use of information here-in in any manner.

Aorta
The main and strongest artery to the heart the aorta carries blood supply
to the system pumped out from the left ventricle.

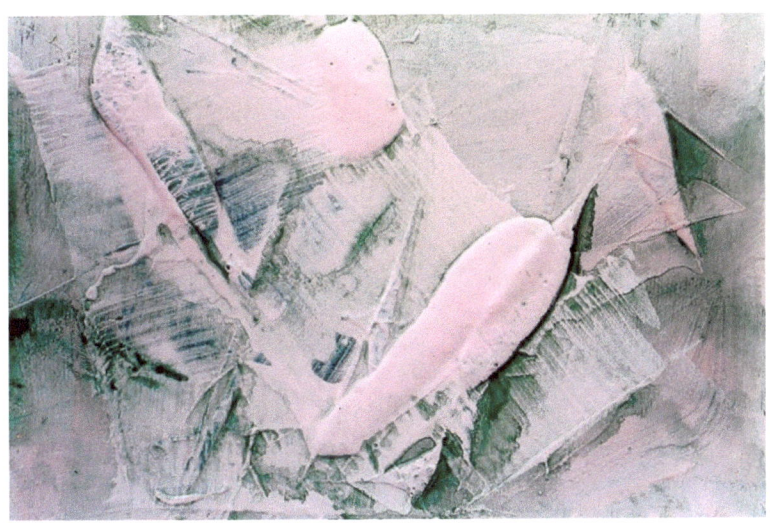

Arch of Atlas
The primary support to the head the Arch of Atlas is a cervical vertebra
with a central and two lateral apertures. The ring of bone is shaped with
an anterior posterior arch and a lateral mass at the junction of these arches.

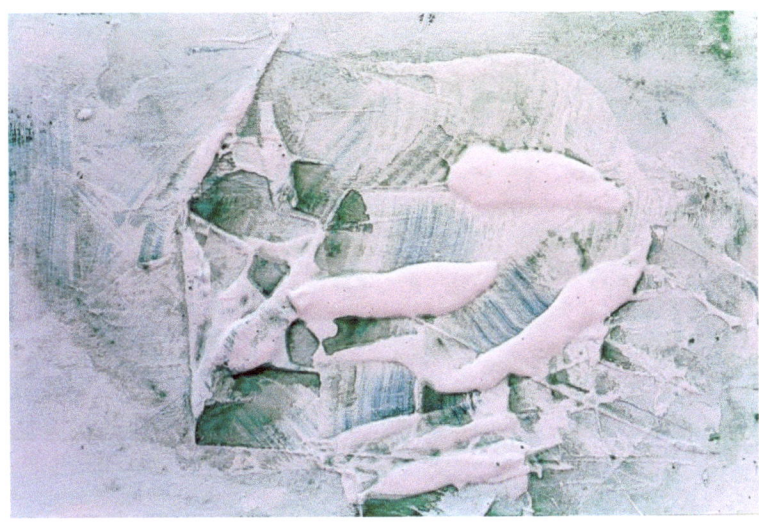

Arm
Manipulative limbs either side of the trunk of the body operates by flexion of muscles in the forearm and upper arm, connected with the scapula and humerus joints of the shoulder.

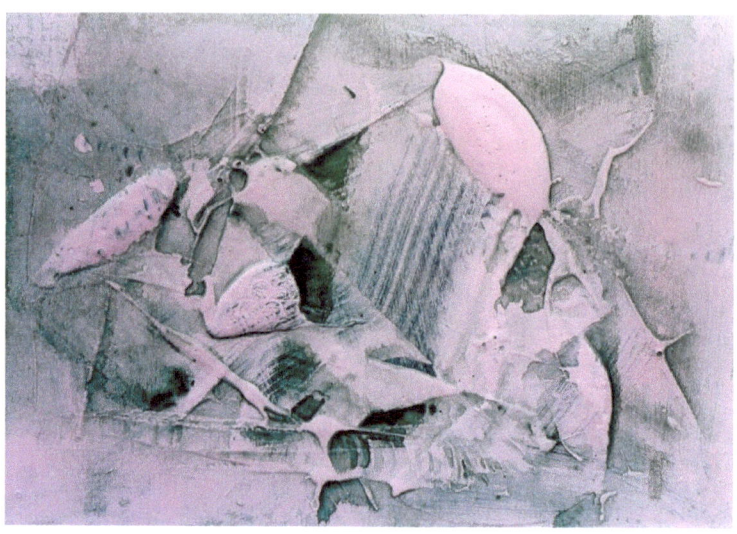

Artery
Branching out from the Aorta arteries act as vehicles for blood circulation away from the heart. They carry oxygen, hormones and nutrients for the system.

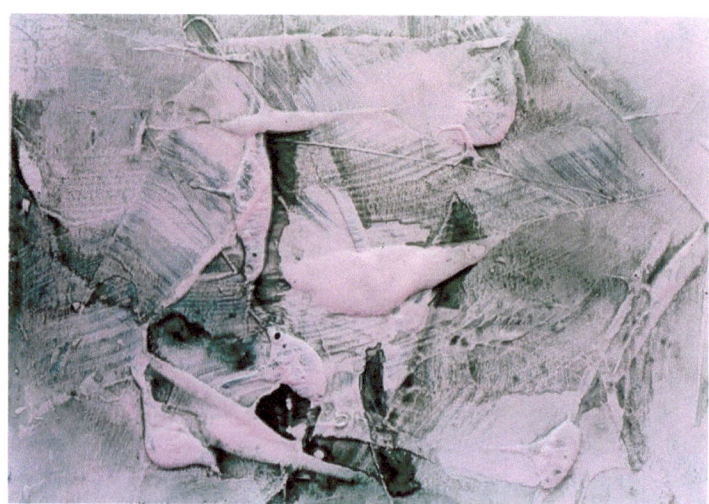

Atrium

The right and left atrium are partitions of the heart, respective compartments through which oxygen-poor blood and oxygen-rich blood is processed.

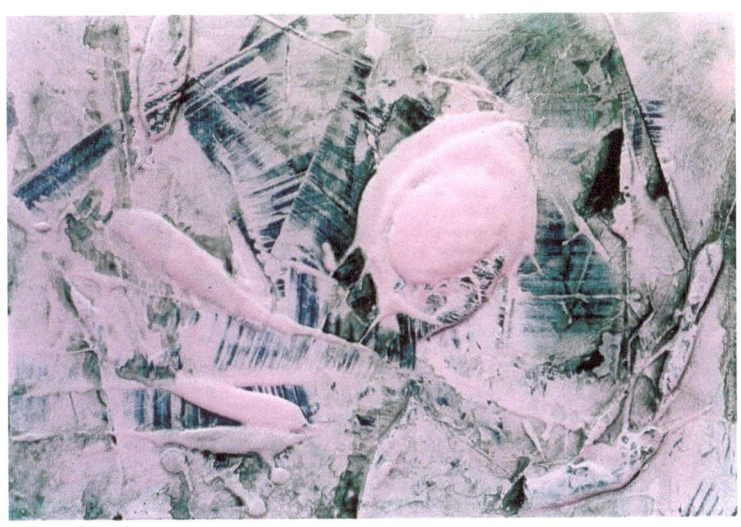

Bladder

An agent in the disposal of waste fluids from the system the bladder is a sac located on the floor of the pelvis. Formed in the kidney urine is carried by theureter to the bladder for storage, from which it is expelled in a process of micturition via the urethra.

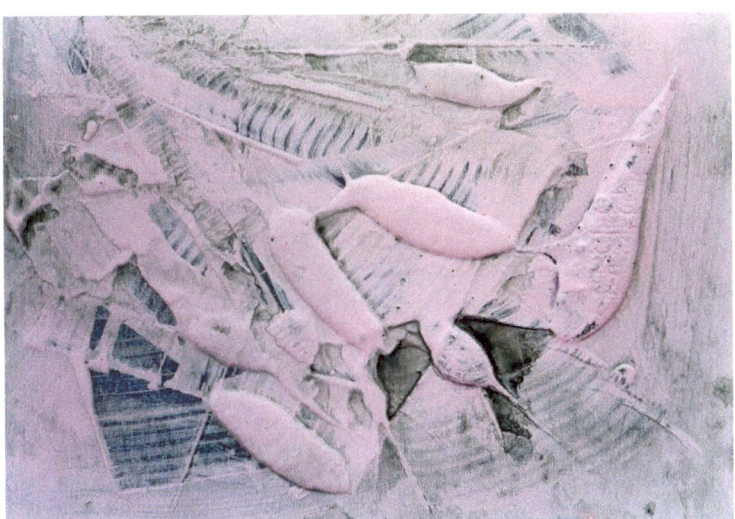

Bones

The skeleton is a framework of two hundred and six bones of varied size and composition.These act as supports for the body, as levers for muscular activity, in protection of organs and soft tissue, and for areas of blood cell development.

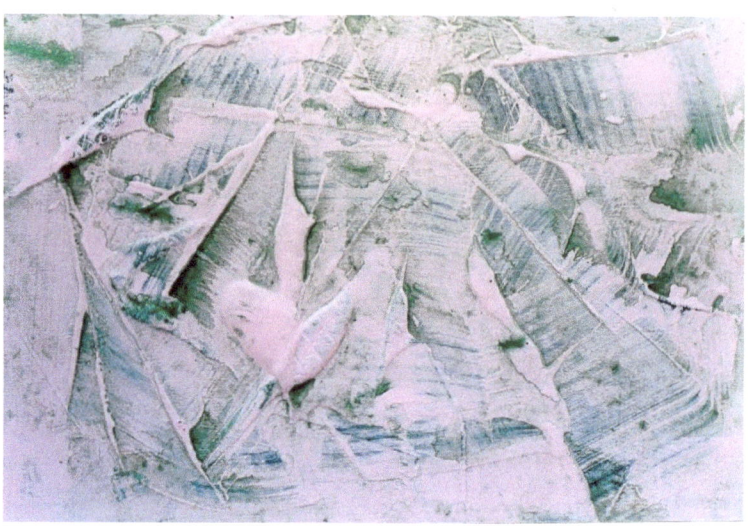

Brain

The central and peripheral nervous systems are governed by a unified network of communication. Brain tissue receives and interprets stimuli which generates specific impulses, instructions for action relayed as sophisticated mental decisions or automatic reflex via the spine.

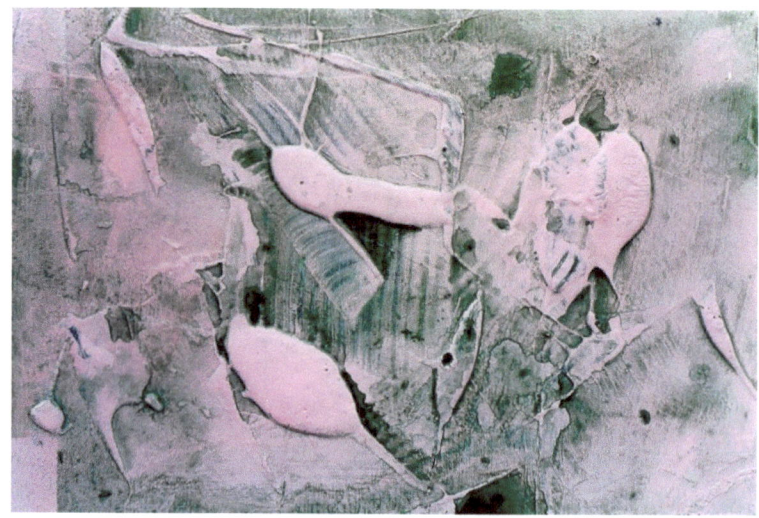

Branches
Membranes described respectively as marginal and circumflex branches on the surface of the heart, and as cochlear and vestibular branches in the ear, extend blood supply and the internal nervous system.

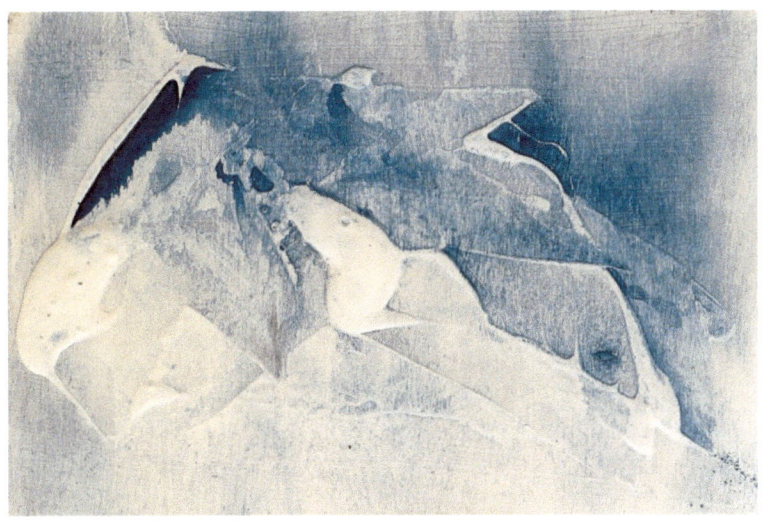

Breast
Female breasts contain mammory glands which process and secrete milk for newborn children. This is regulated by hormones and prolactin within thepituitary gland. The opening of the mammory gland is located at thepigmented circle of the aureola

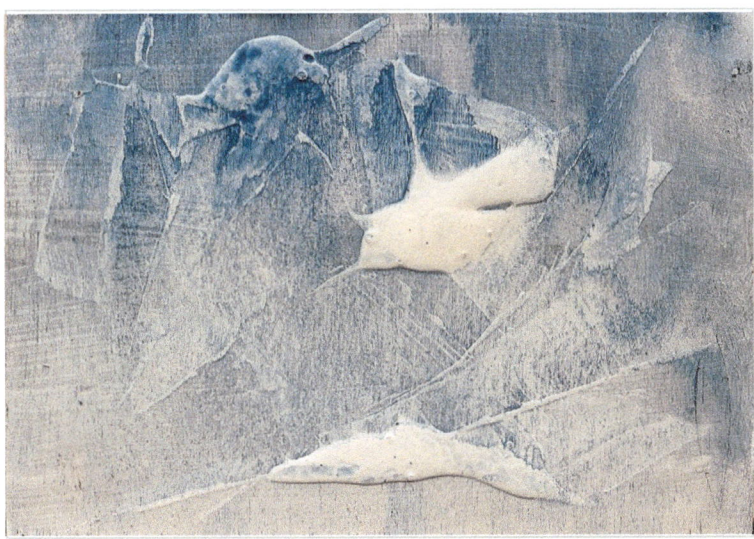

Bronchi

The left and right Bronchus are the respiratory passages which lead from the Trachea. These extend in tree form into the air sacs of the lungs.

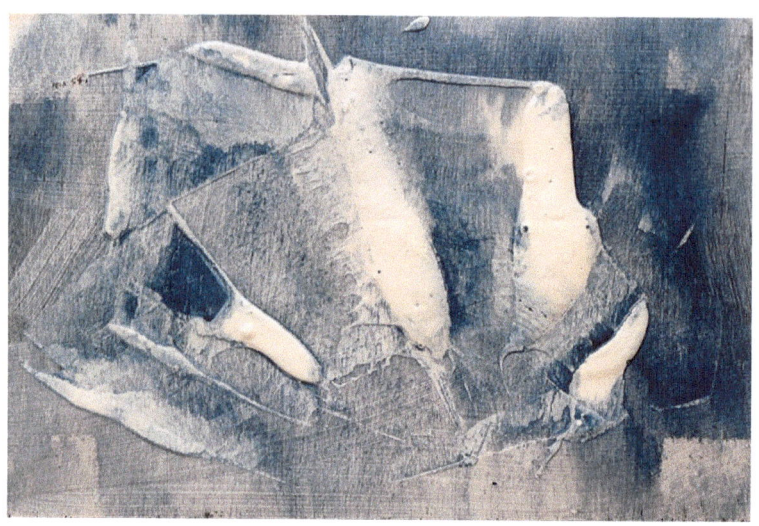

Bulb

A structure attached to the surface of the urogenital diaphragm is enclosed by spongy muscle, and is found within the root of the male penis.

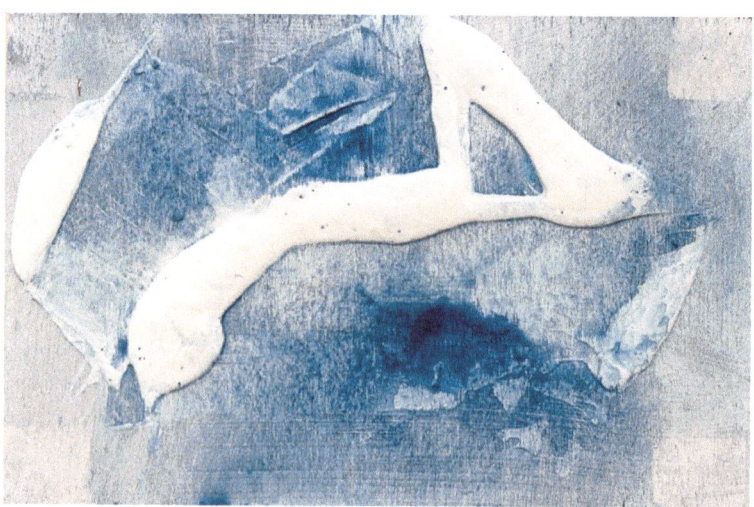

Buttocks

The structure of the posterior is imposed on the upper thigh muscles, dividing in the cleft surface of buttocks. The size of the gluteus maximus muscle of the buttock varies in male and female according to their differing pelvic frame size and load bearing dynamic.

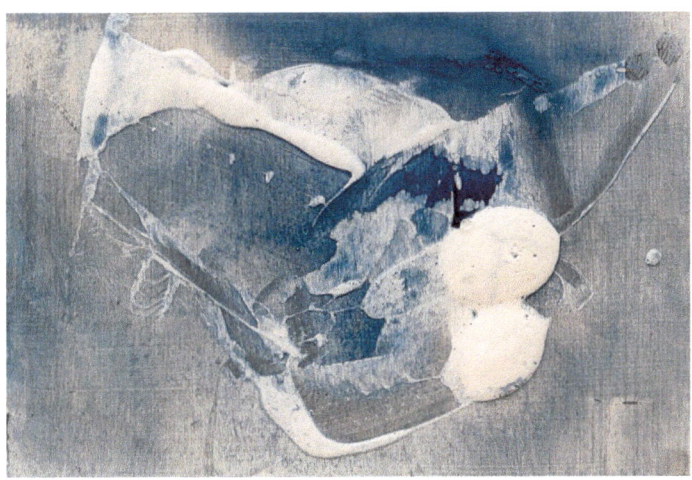

Canal

A duct or passage in varied parts such as the inner ear (lateral and anterior canal), or anus (anal canal)

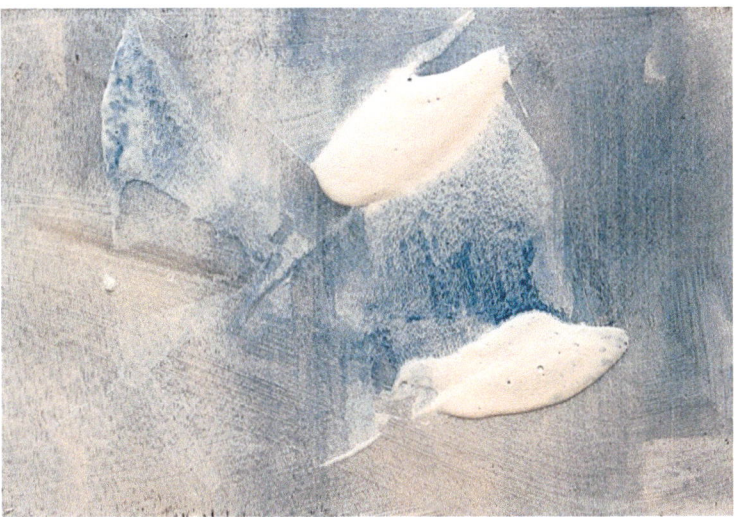

Capillary
A stem like duct such as the peritubular capillary of the kidney which filters blood flow through the system.

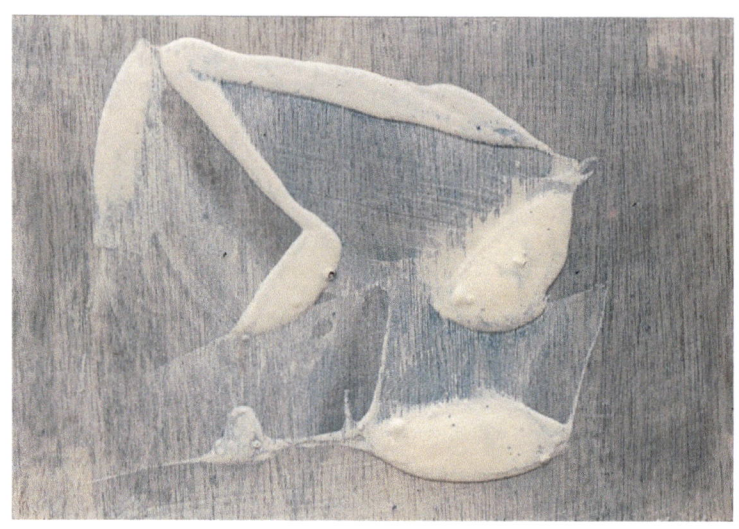

Cartilage
An inner and outer fibrous layer which absorbs impact to joints of bones, and eases friction at their point of conjunction.

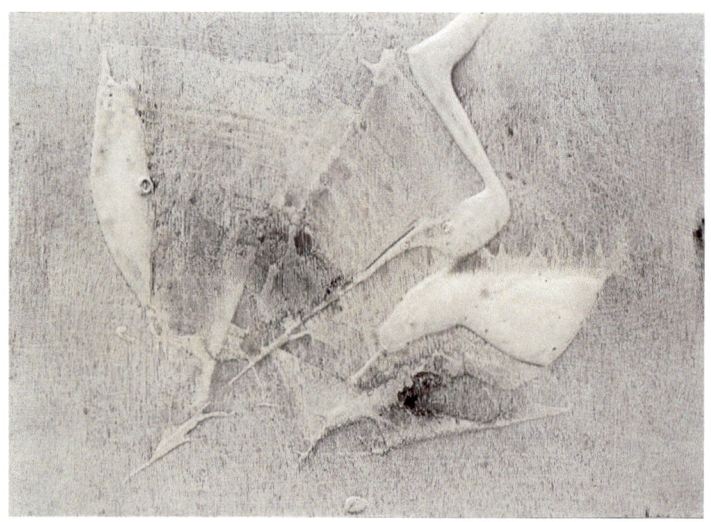

Cavity

Chambers known as cavities exist throughout the body to
house and protect internal organs of varied size and shape.

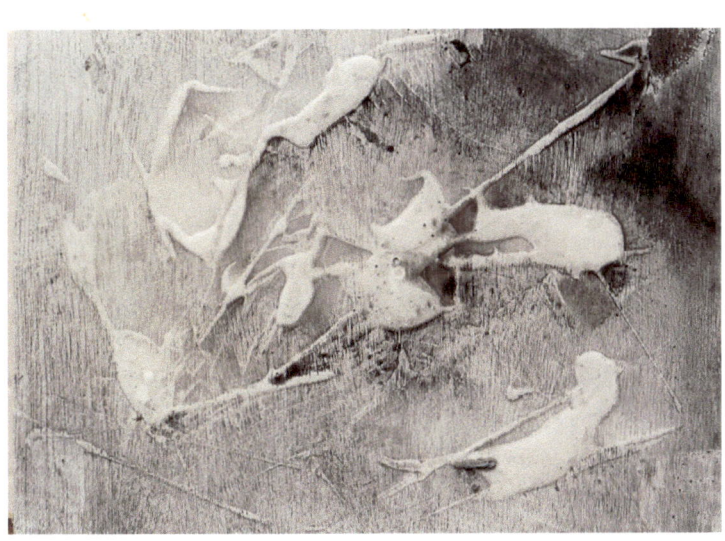

Cells

The core unit of active life within the human physical system,
the cell contains a collection of varied biochemical mechanisms
enclosed within a membrane layer. Cells cannot be typified as they assume
multiple forms and function within different parts of the body.

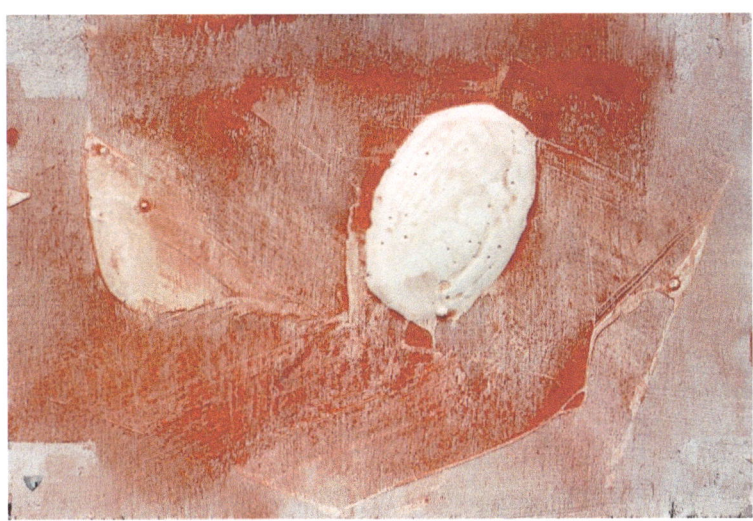

Cerebellum

A divided mass of neural tissue the cerebellum is supported by the posterior aspect of the skull. Composed of three lobes: the anterior, posterior and flocculonodular lobes, it is linked by nerve tracts to other parts of the brain. Impulses received from the spinal cord are filtered through

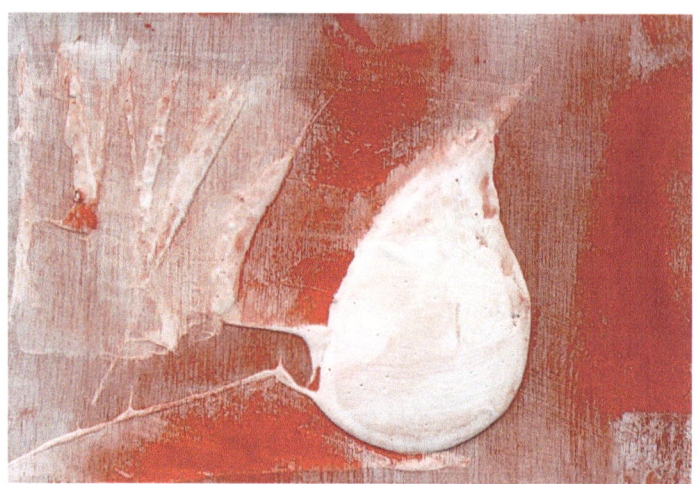

Cervix

Found in the female reproductive system the cervix is a narrow opening which leads from the vagina to the uterus.

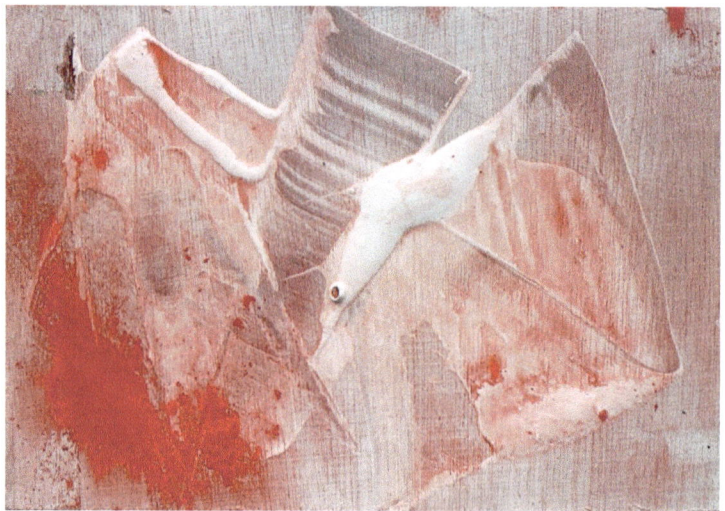

Column

The spinal column is composed of twenty six bones; twenty four vertebrae with the coccyx and sacrum. The column of vertebral discs shields the spinal cord and is mapped in five divisions, to the neck-cervical vertebrae, the chest-thoracic vertebrae, lower back-lumbar and sacrum.

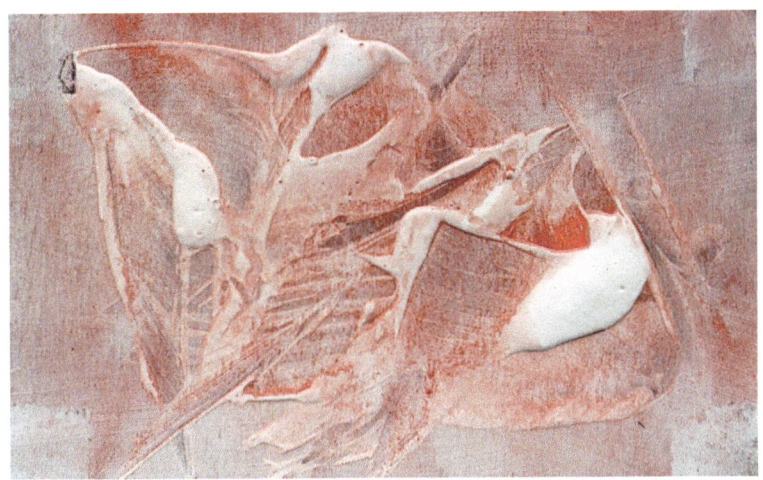

Conchae

Ridged bones in the respiratory tracts of the nose, the superior, middle and inferior nasal concha are covered with a vascular mucus.

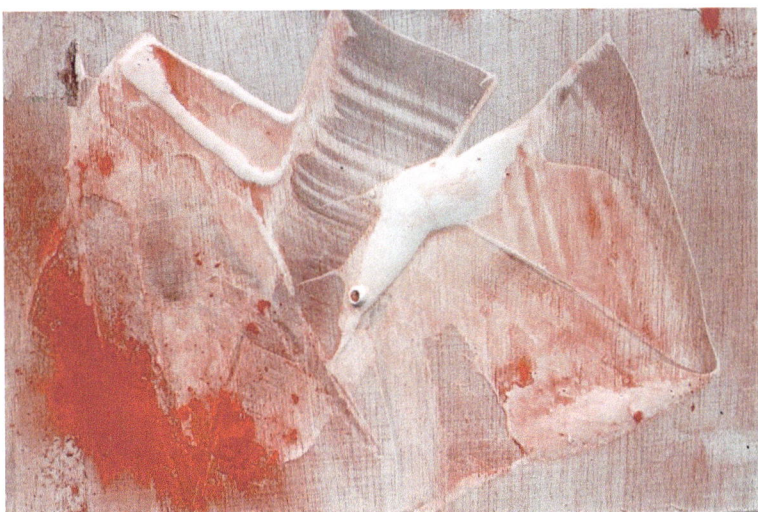

Cornea
A transparent layer of the eye the cornea assists the focus of light
as it passes through the pupil, cornea and lens to the retina.

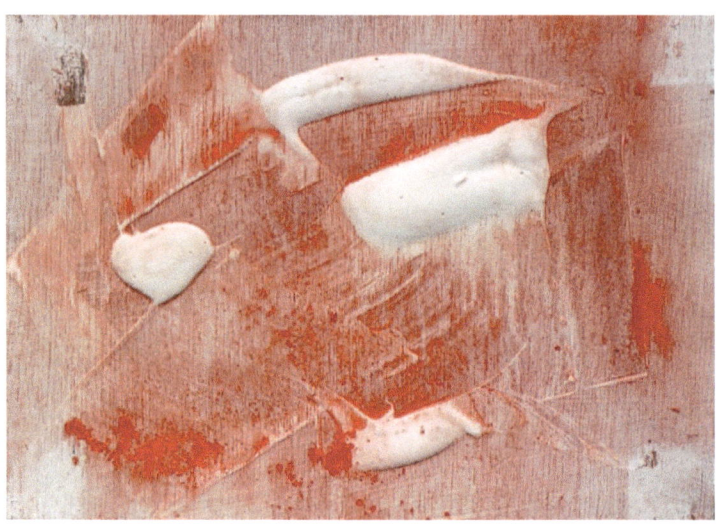

Cuneiform
Situated in the distal row of the foot the medial, intermediate and lateral
cuneiform link the navicular joint with the shafts of the metatarsals.

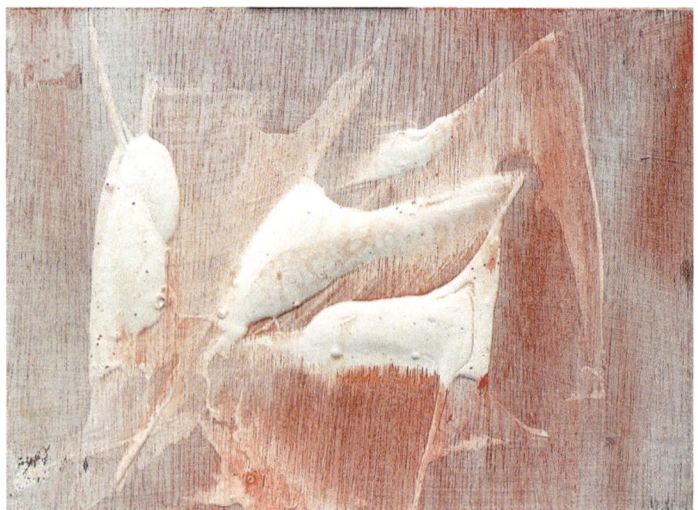

Diaphragm
The dome-shaped muscle of the diaphragm expands to permit air to the lungs. Anchored by strong ligaments it forms the floor of the thoracic cavity.

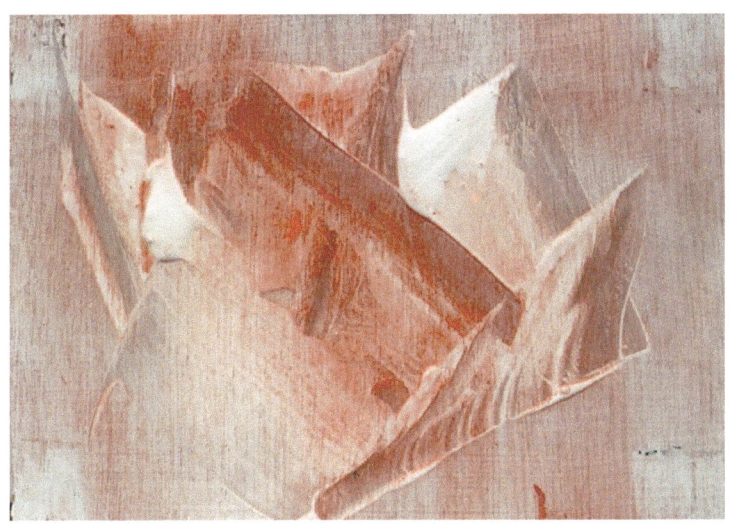

Digits
Individual bones that form the phalanges (fingers) of the hand

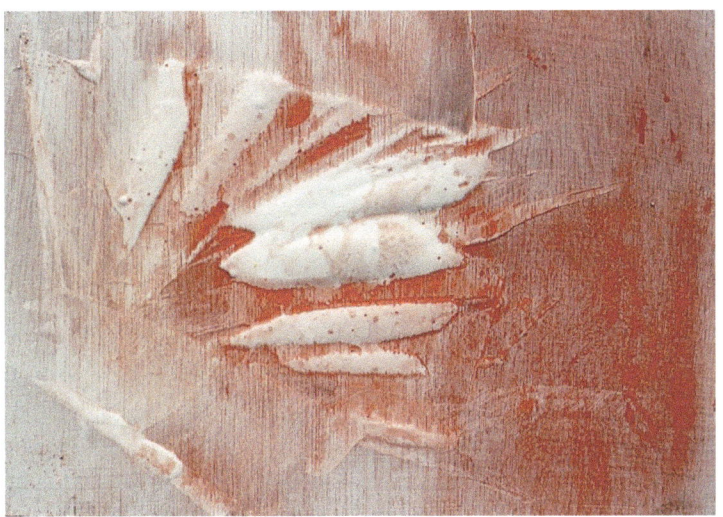

Disks
A fibrous pad of cartilage cushions sections of vertebrae (intervertebral disksof the spinal column,), the pelvic girdle or the forearm and lower leg.

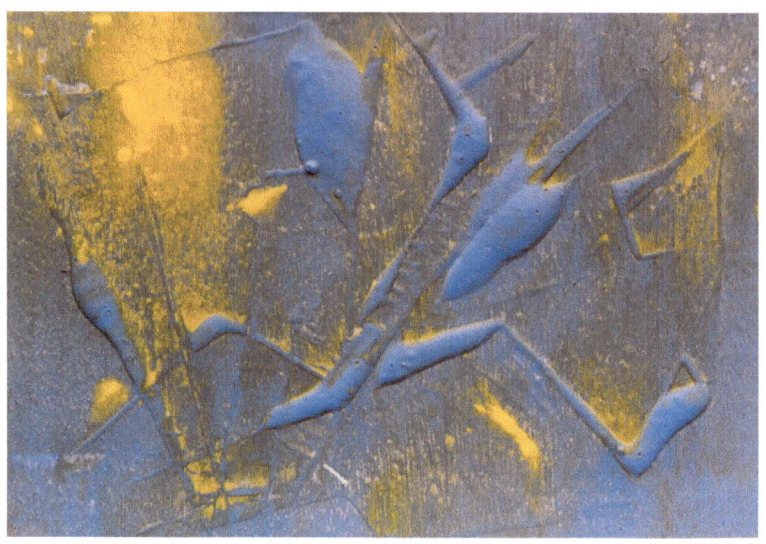

Ducts
Passages for drainage of digested materials from the liver (common bile ducts),enzymes and ions from the pancreas to duodenum. Ejaculatory ducts carry secretions

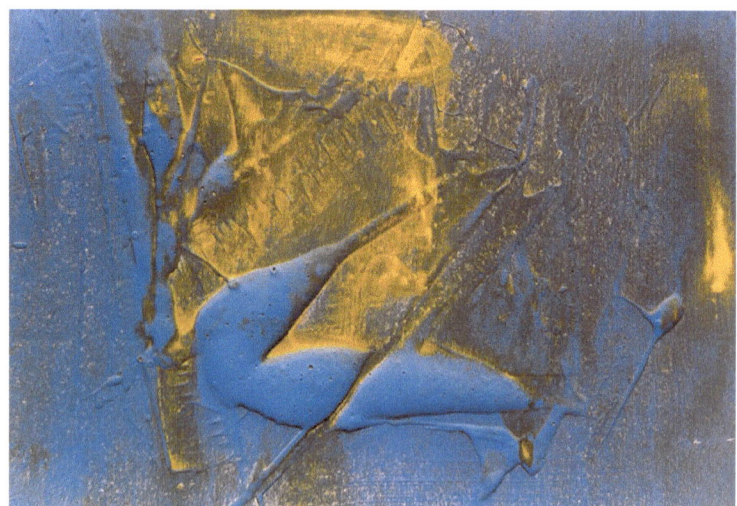

Duodenum

The first part of the small intestine the duodenum receives digested materials emptied from the stomach via the pyloric sphincter.

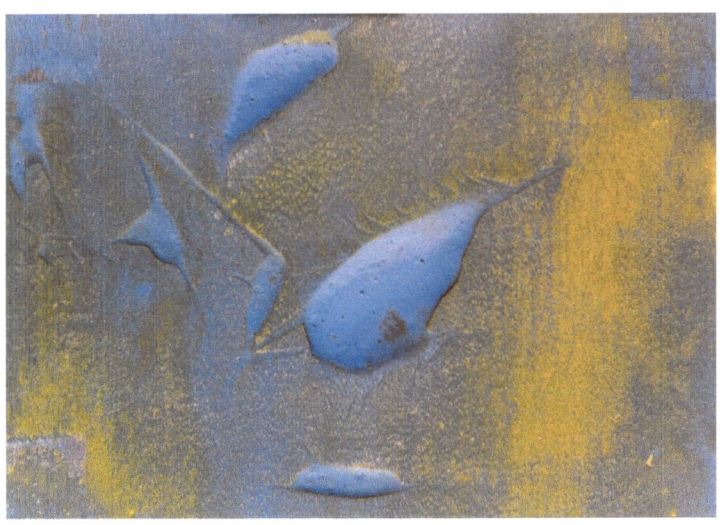

Ear

Governs hearing and balance in the body, sending sensory impulses from received vibrations to the cerebral cortex for interpretation. Receptors for balance and hearing are contained in different sites of the ear.

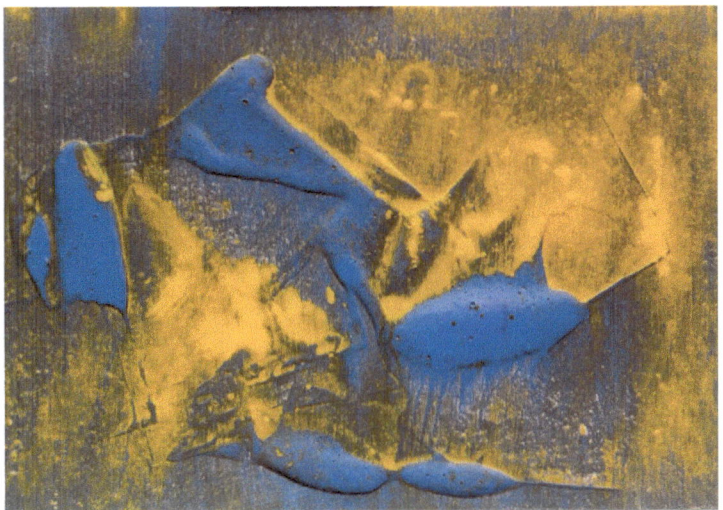

Esophagus
A muscular tube for transport of food to the stomach.

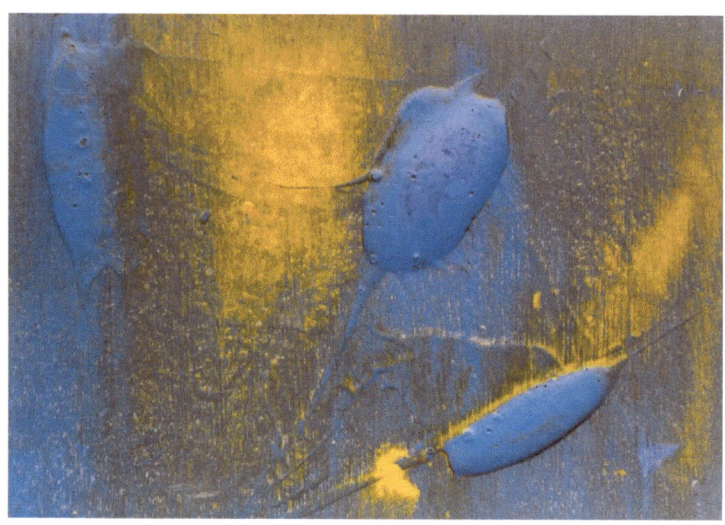

Fascia
A fibrous protective tissue that surrounds the kidney (renal fascia) and the male testes (two layers called the external and internal spermatic fascia)

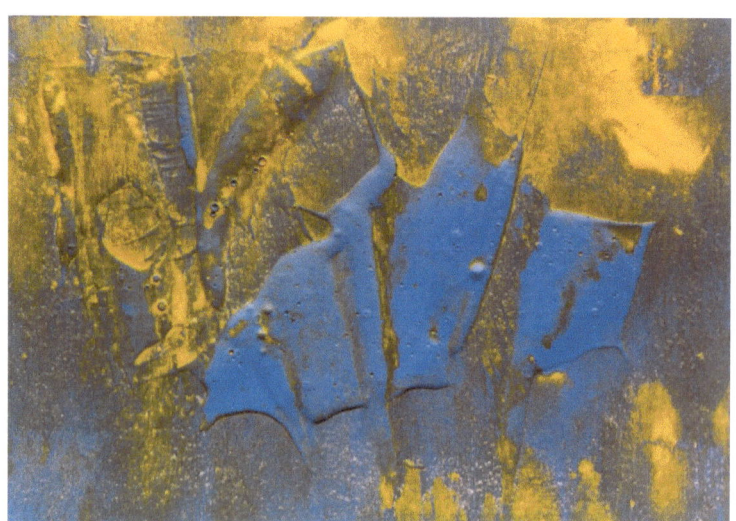

Femur
The thigh bone which extends from the pelvic girdle to the lower leg.

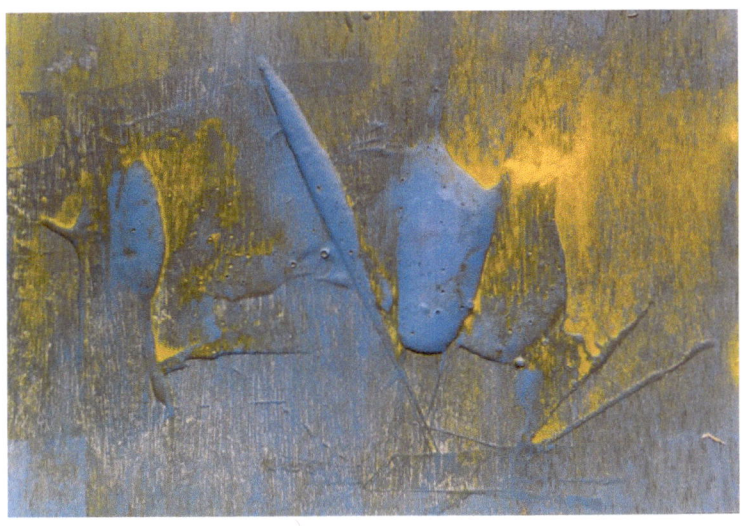

Fibula
One of two lower leg bones the lighter fibula is set beside the tibia, extending from the patella to the tarsals of the ankle.

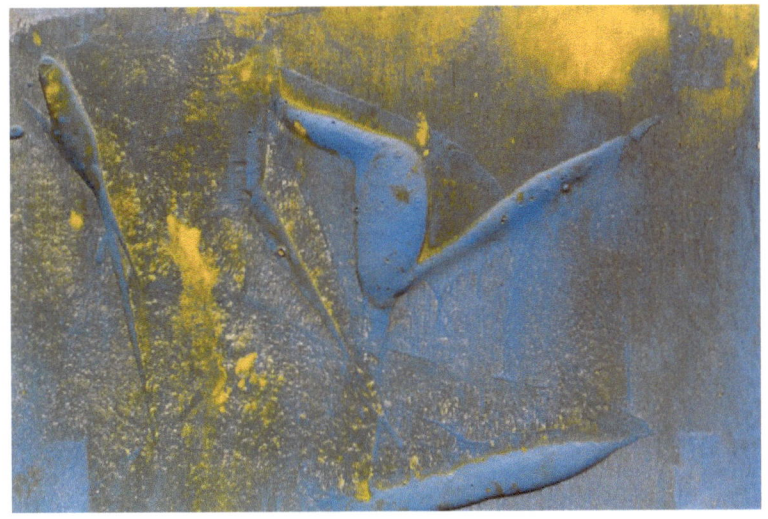

Finger
Extensions of the hand contain a four fingers and a thumb.
Flexible digits in the metacarpals and phalanges allow
basic motions of grasping and balance.

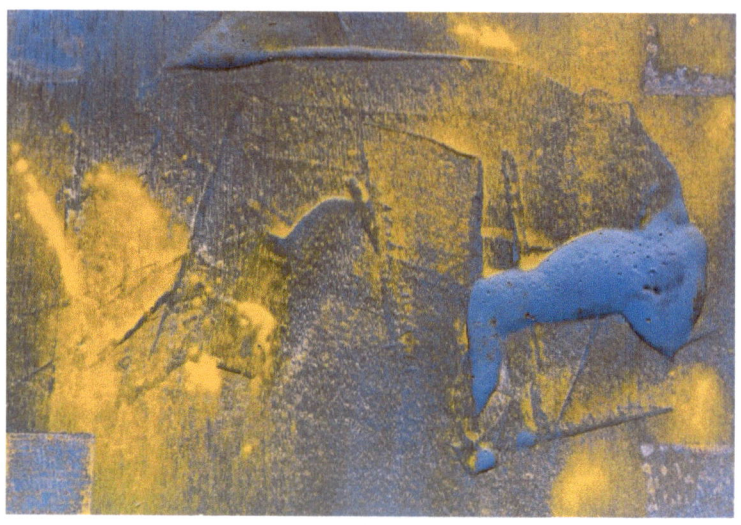

Fissure
A deep groove which divides the hemispheres of the brain,
running from the posterior to anterior lobes of the cerebral cortex.

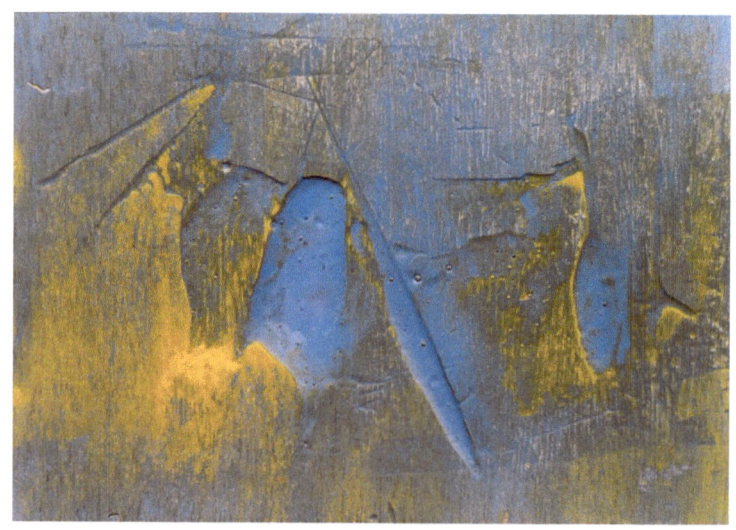

Follicle

Clustered lymphocytes known as follicles occupy the cortex area of the lymph node, acting as part of the immune system.

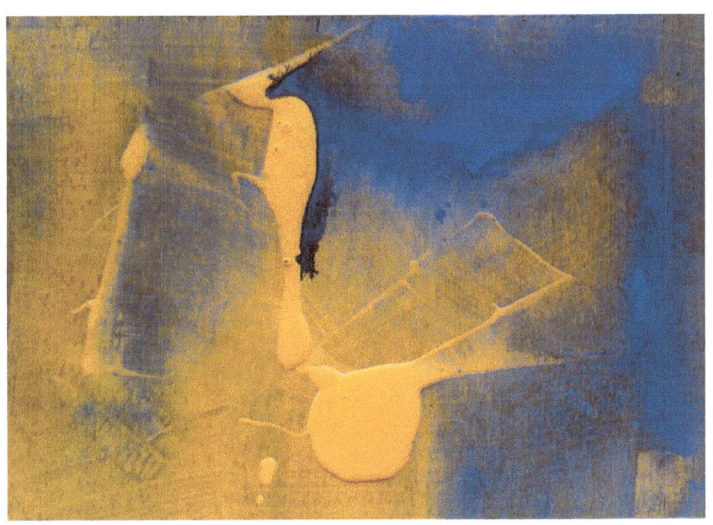

Foot

The agent for walking and balance the foot, like the hand, is composed of twenty six bones. The three regions of the foot include the tarsus, metatarsus and the phalanges.

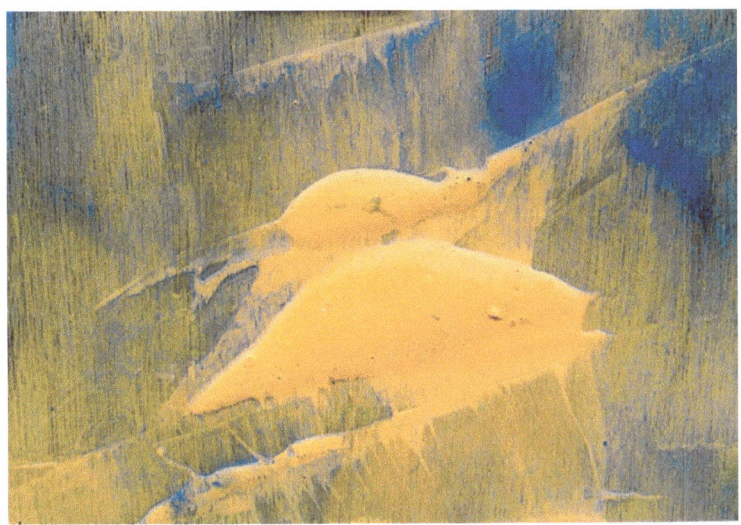

Gland
A cellular structure the gland is designed to synthesize and produce a secretion. Described as endocrine and ductless if distributed to a blood vessel, ex-ocrineand ducted glands deliver mucous, oil and saliva, to specific body parts.

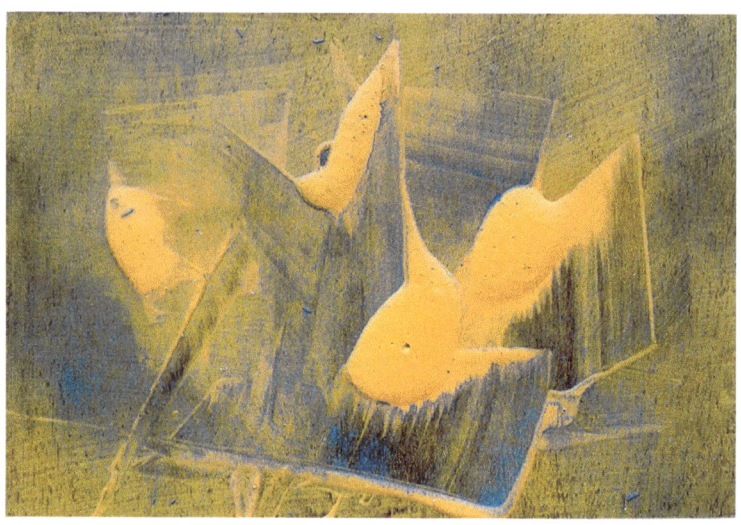

Gonadotropins
Hormones which are influential in the cycle of reproduction, gonadotropins stimulate follicles.

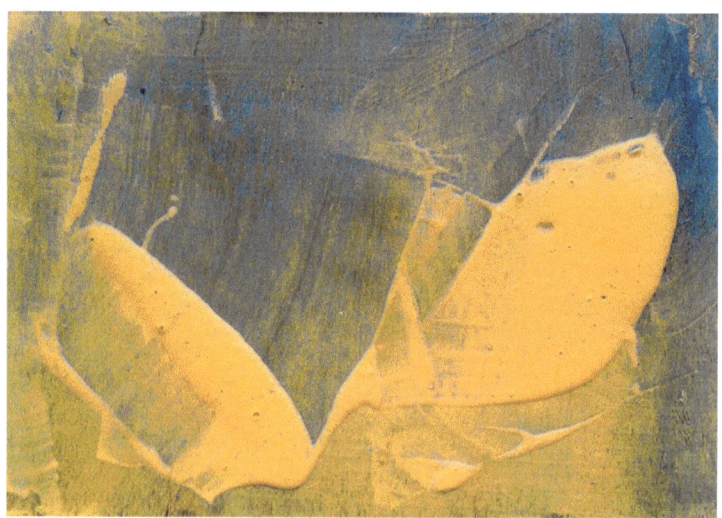

Heart
The central pump to the physical system, the heart receives blood and contracting, propels it through two closed circuits, supplying body cells organs and tissues, and to the lungs. Blood returns to the heart after use via the superior and inferior vena cava.

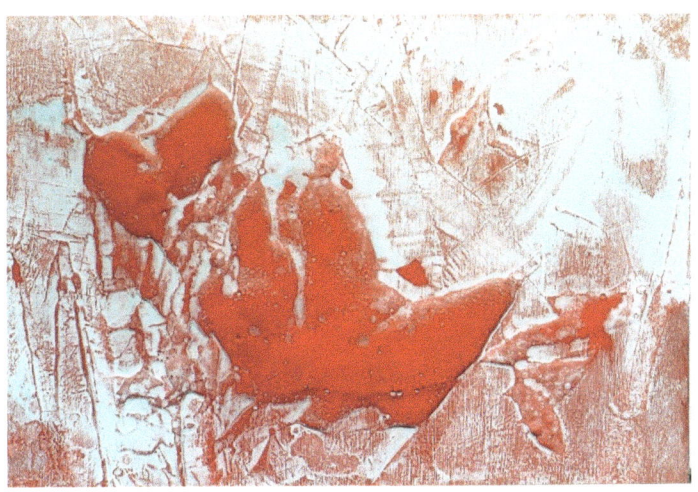

Heel
The heel of the foot is called calcaneus. The achilles (calcaneal) tendon bonds the calf muscle to the heel.

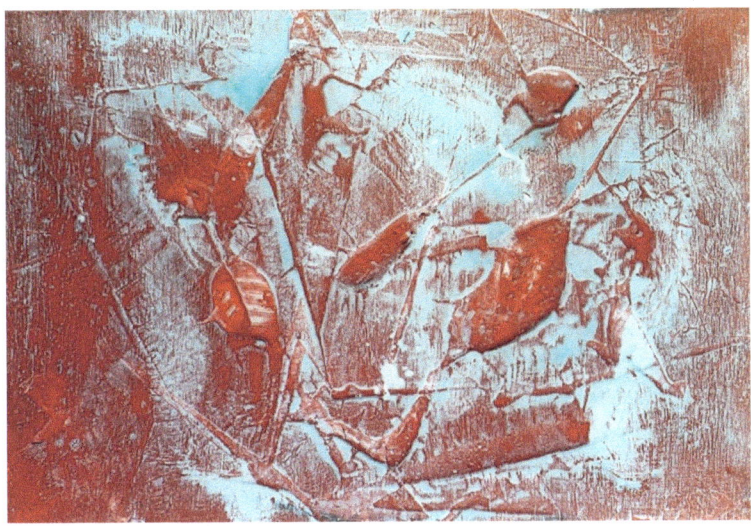

Hip
The lateral aspect of the pelvic girdle the hip is more pronounced in weight in the female than the male. It heads the long bone of the upper leg (femur).

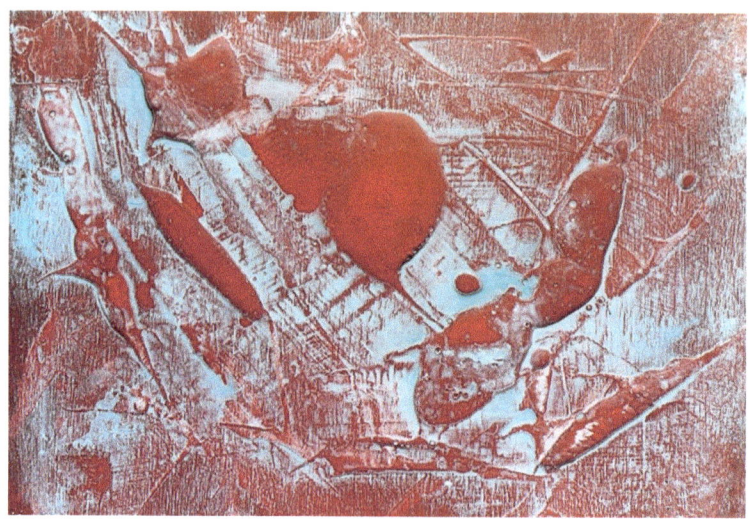

Intestine
Receiving material from the stomach the digestive process continues in the twenty feet winding pipe of the small intestine, agent of absorpton of nutrients.

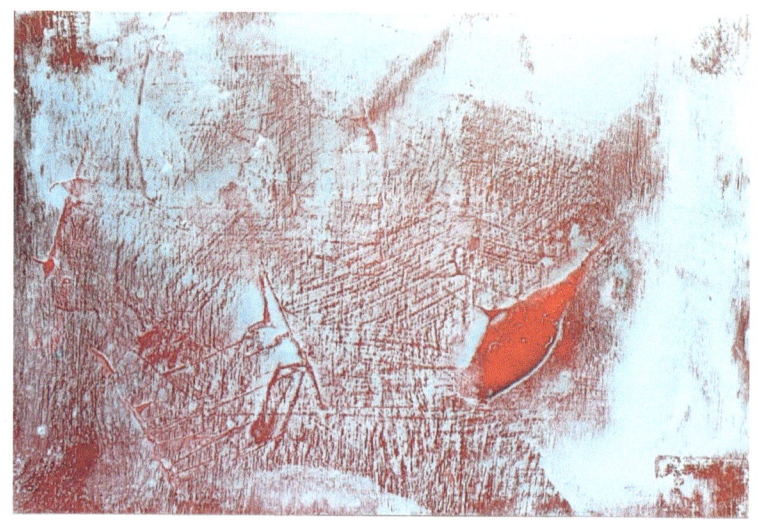

Iris

Beyond the cornea is the coloured aspect of the iris. It expands and closes by muscular movement allowing filtration of perceived light to the pupil.

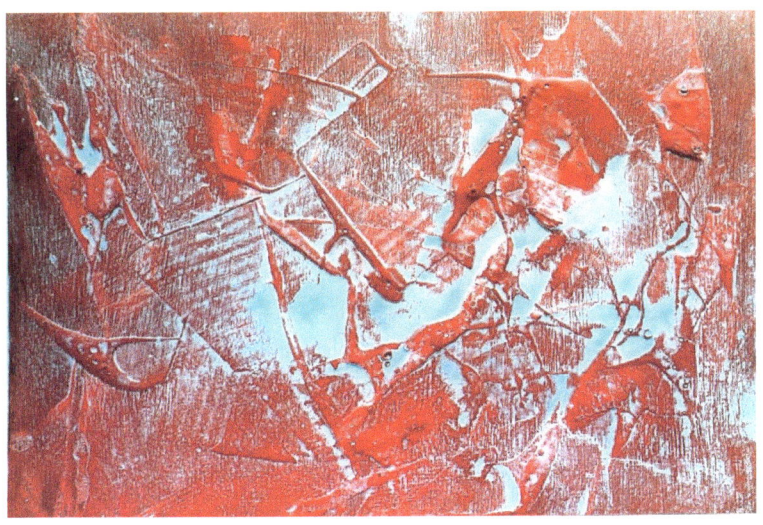

Jaw

The jawbone (mandible) is situated in the lower aspect of the face, joined theskull at the middle ear. Powerful muscles and tendons such as the masseter and temporalis act in concert for biting and grinding.

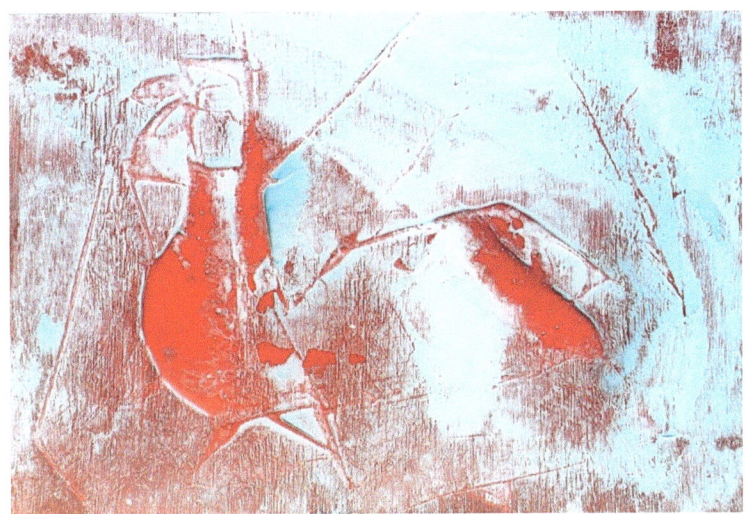

Knee

Located at the extent of the long bone of the upper leg where it joins to the tibia. The small wedge shaped sesamoid bone is embedded in tendons of the knee which it protects.

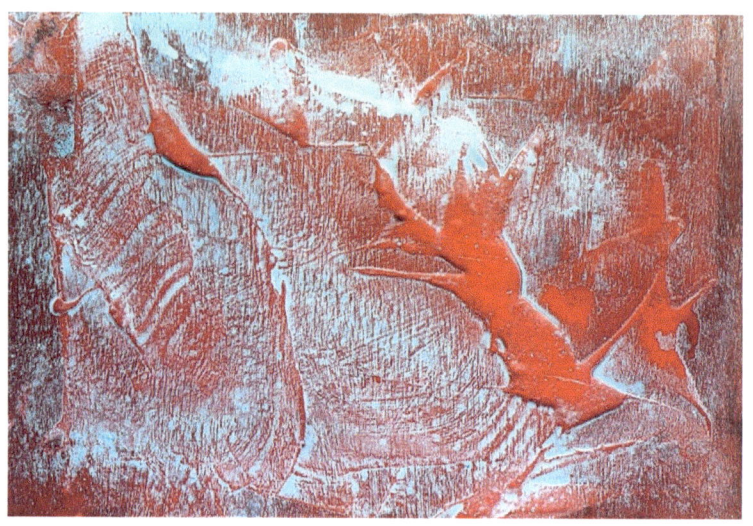

Knuckle

The prominent head of the metacarpals, called knuckles in the hand, articulates with the phalanges, the first section of bones in the fingers.

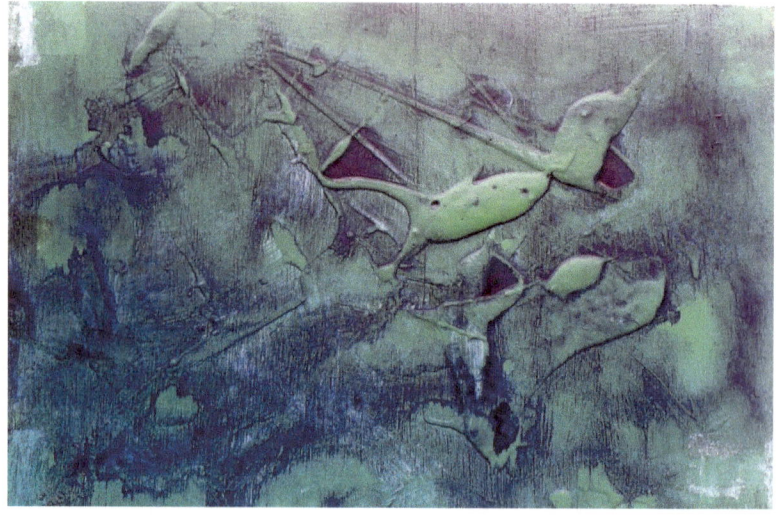

Labia
The labia form the entrance to the female reproductive system;
the pair of labia majora (external cover) and labia minora,
the internal fold of the vulva.

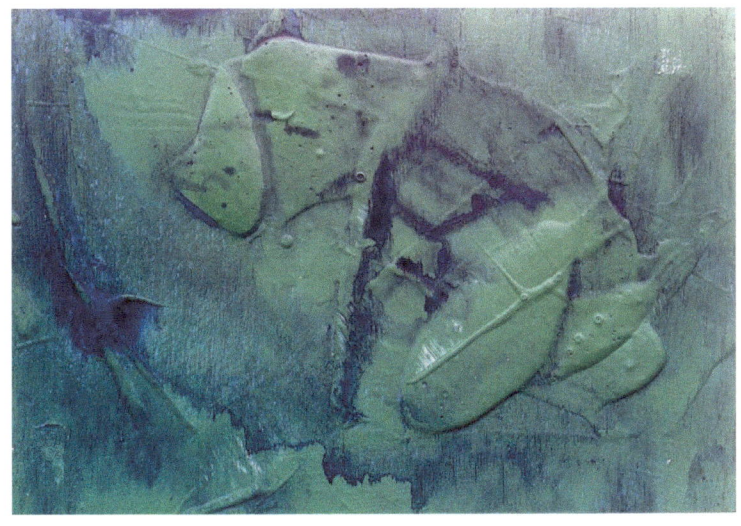

Labyrinth
Forming a passage within the inner ear the labyrinth
consistes of two layers, the outer bony and the inner membraneous.
These are interspersed by perilymph fluid.

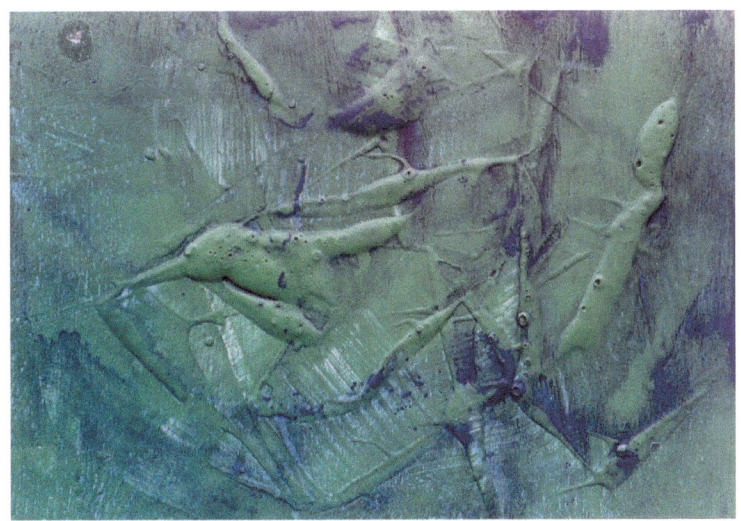

Lung
The pair of air sacs situated within the thoracic cavity of the ribcage. Expanded and contracted by the intercostal muscles and the diaphragm, lungs act for oxygen exchange within the respiratory system.

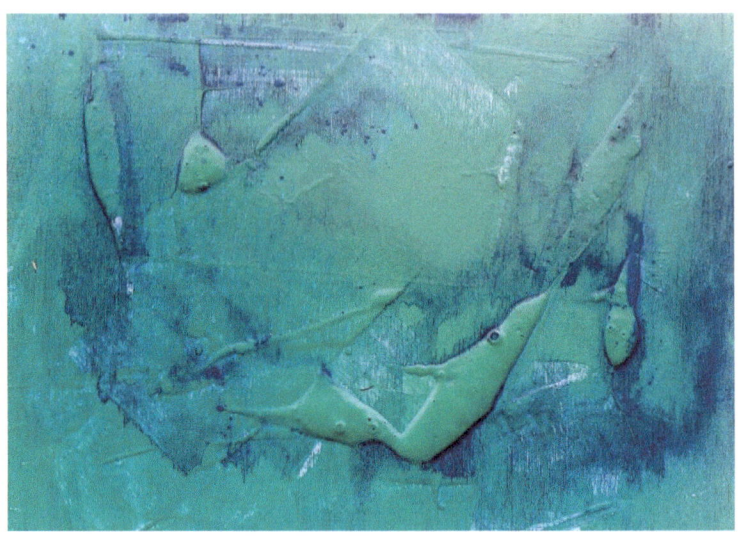

Metatarsal
The long bones of the foot connected with the cuneiform of the upper end and the phalanges of the toes.

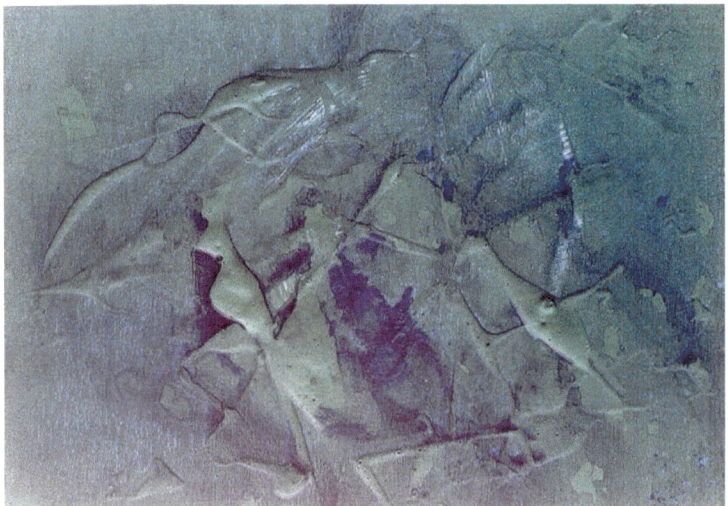

Mouth
The recepticle for food and liquid intake, and chamber of articulation of sound.

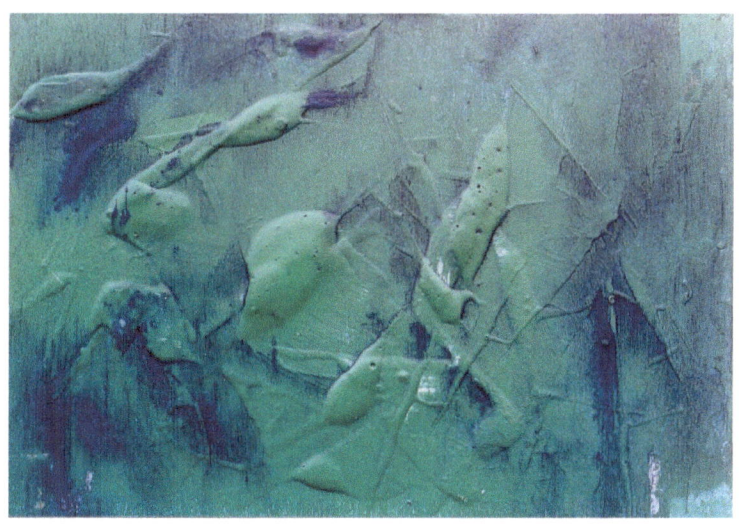

Neck
The support to the head, the neck set at the height of the spinal column connected to the cranium. It is composed of superficial muscles of support (sternocleidomastoid) and deep muscles of the throat

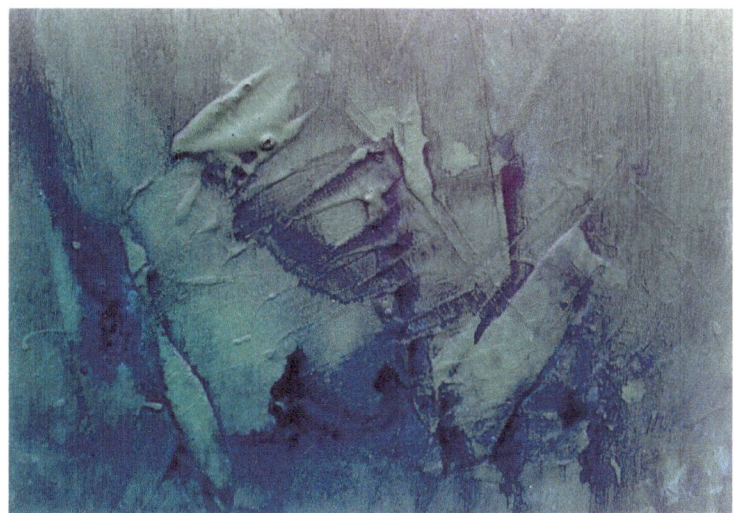

Nucleus

The nucleus determines the genetic pattern of individual cells and is at the core of their activity.

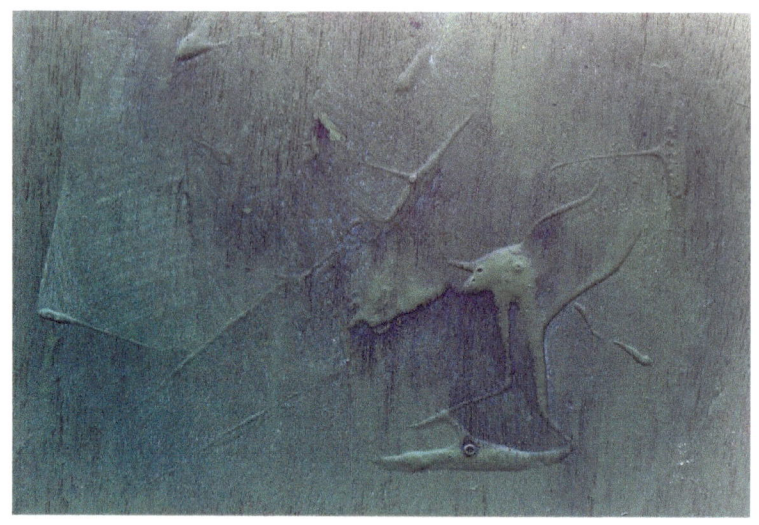

Orifice

An opening, internal in the ureter (bladder) or external to the vagina.

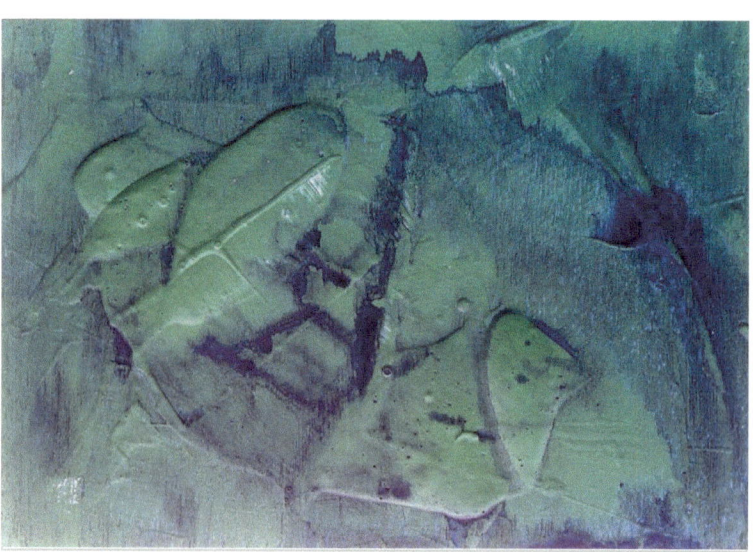

Pelvis

The supporting frame to the hips and torso the pelvic girdle is of a broader span in the female than the male. The pelvic bones meet with the apex of the spinal column (sacrum) at the sacroiliac joint.

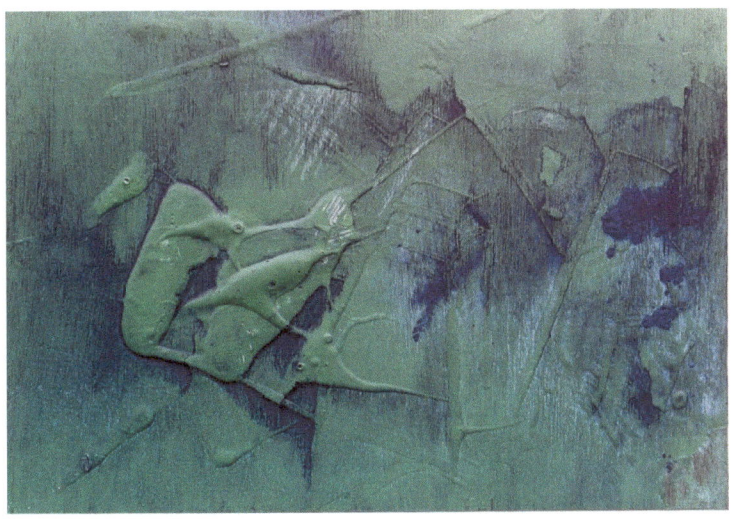

Perineum

The floor of the pelvic diaphragm, mapped from the sacrum and coccyx to the ischium and pubis, is called the perineum.
Muscular structures correspond in male and female, which are active in controlledevacuation of digested material through the urethra and anus.

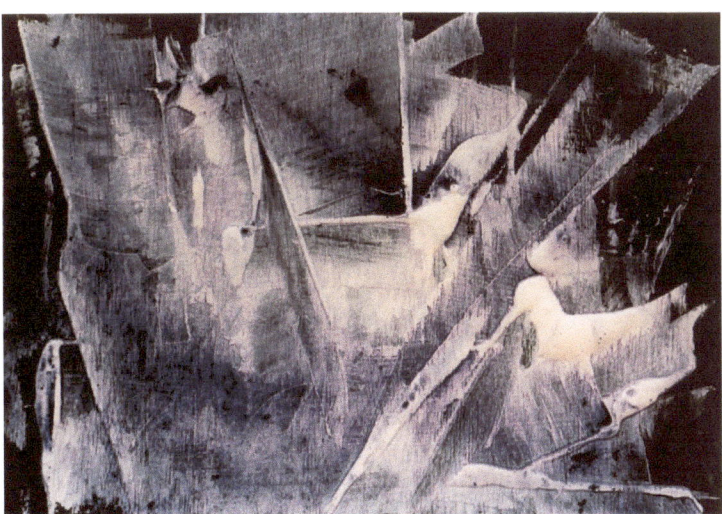

Pigment
A layer of cells in the eye which absorbs and prevents reflection of stray light. Also a constituent of skin surface which affects its colour and tone.

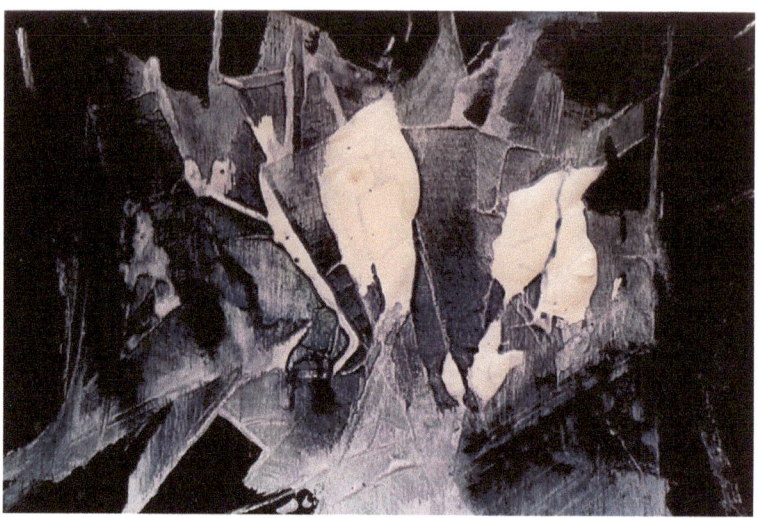

Pubis
The frontal aspect of the pelvic girdle determined as an arch. It is wider in the female, greater than 90° extent, than the male, less than 90°.

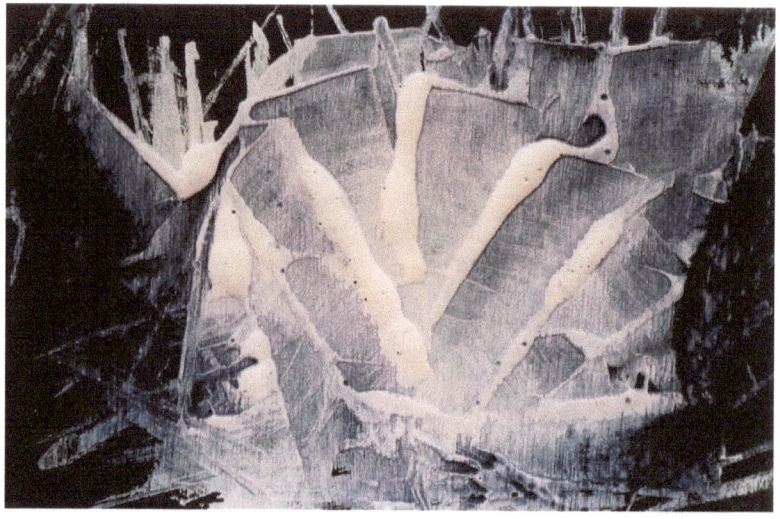

Rectum

The chamber of storage for waste material from the body lies behind the wall of the cervix in the female, and the prostatic urethra in the male, and above the anus.

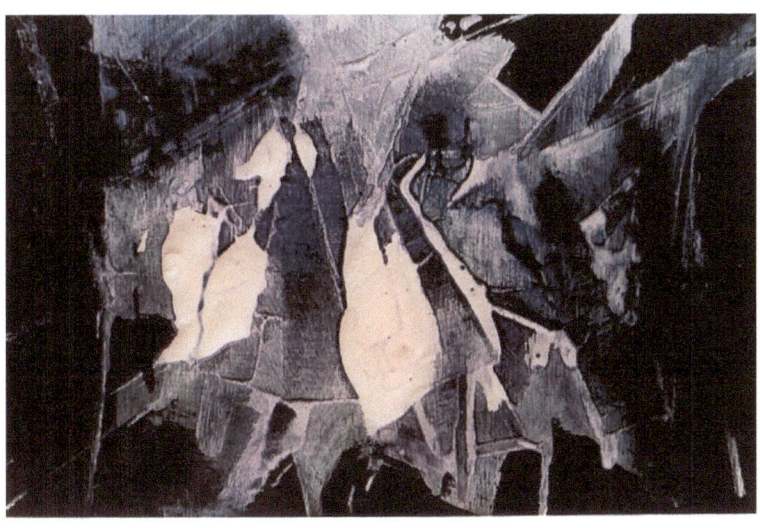

Retina

Light passes through the pupil cornea and lens to the wall of the retina (neural tunic). The external surface of the eye, known as the outer retina,

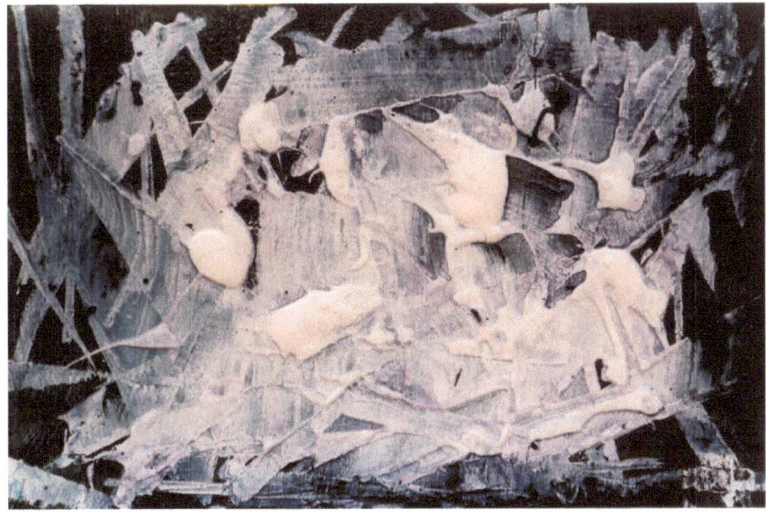

Rib Cage

The ribcage (thoracic cage) contains a rack of sternum and costal cartilages joined at the rear to vertebrae of the spine. Composed of true, false and floating ribs,

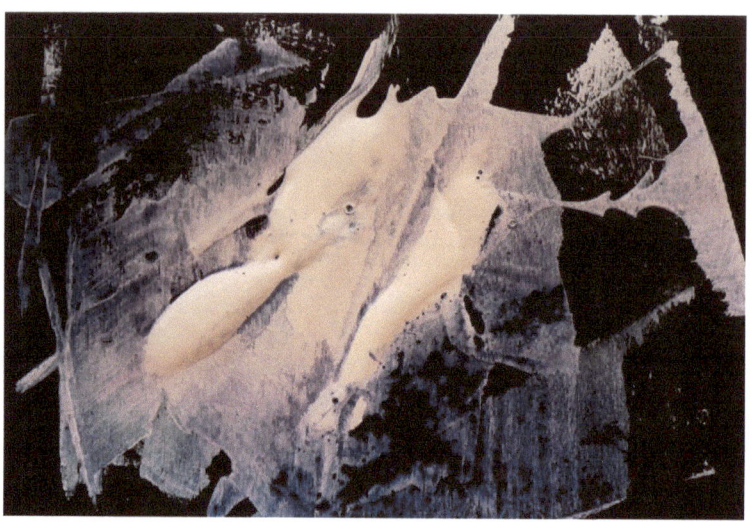

Sacrum

Situated at the lower extent of the spine the sacrum connects the vertebral column with the pelvic girdle. Its substantial construction is designed to meet the considerable pressures of body weight which bear down on the lumbar region.

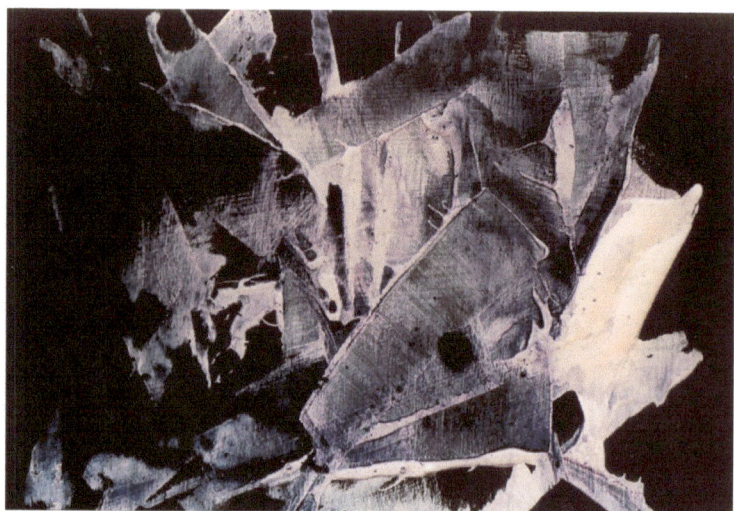

Scalp
Covering the external surface of the head, the scalp consists of an outer (endosteal) layer and an inner layer, interspersed with blood and soft tissue.

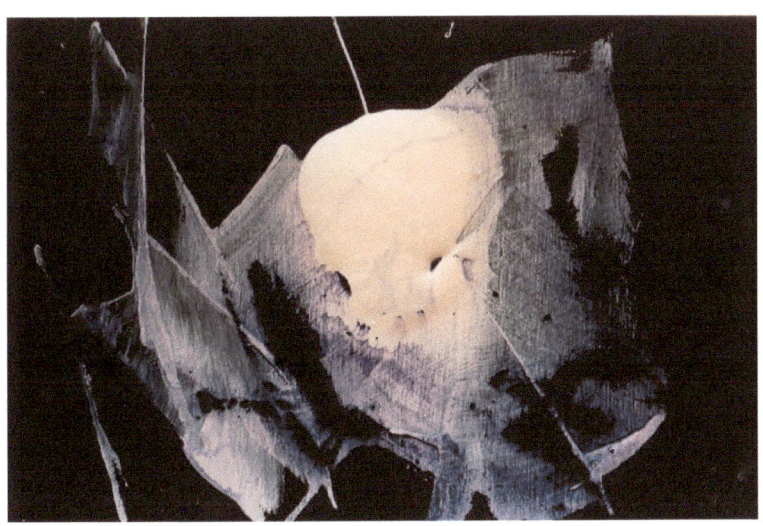

Shin
The external aspect of the ankle bones (tarsals) including the heel of the foot.

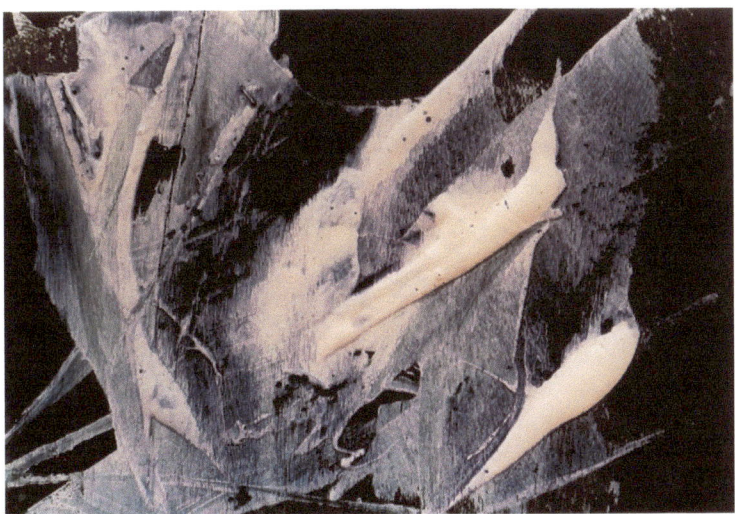

Shoulder

The frame of the shoulder conjoins the bones of the arms (Humerus) at the collar bone (clavicle), and to the shoulder blades (scapula). The powerful deltoid and trapezius muscles protect and support the abdominal organs, the spine and the ribcage.

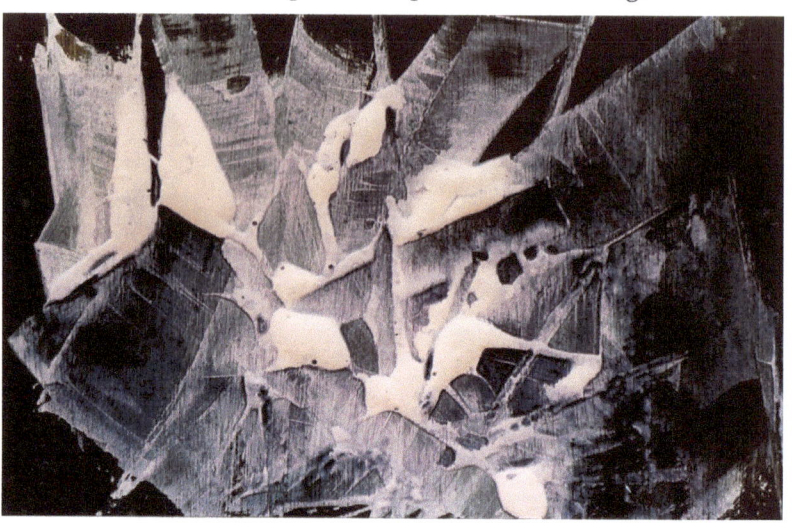

Skin

A protective tissue covering the entire body, skin (integument) is composed of three layers, the outer (epidermis), middle (dermis), and subcutaneous (hypodermis). The external surface allows hair growth, and shields againstemperature, light and chemical invasion. The internal lyer (stratum basale) transmutes by a process of mytosis to superficial layer cells.

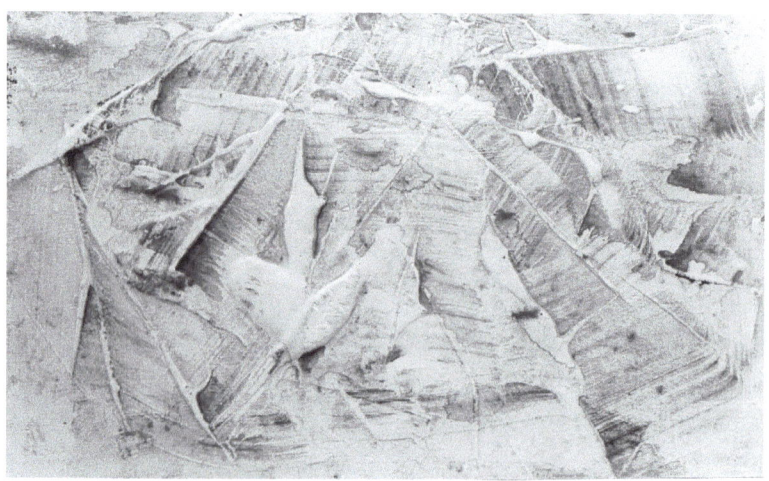

Skull
The bony structure of the head protects the brain, eyes and mouth, and internal organs of the ear. It is composed of the cranium (dome), face and jaw (mandible). It is supported by the neck and the vertebral column of the spine.

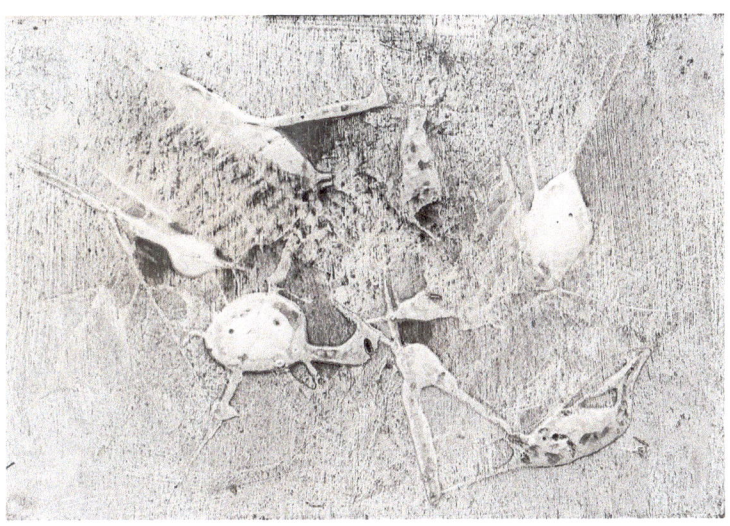

Spine
The vertebral column of the spine enclosing the spinal nerve, extends from the Arch of Atlas down to the sacrum and coccyx, and the pelvic girdle. Its twenty four vertebrae are cushioned by intervertebral

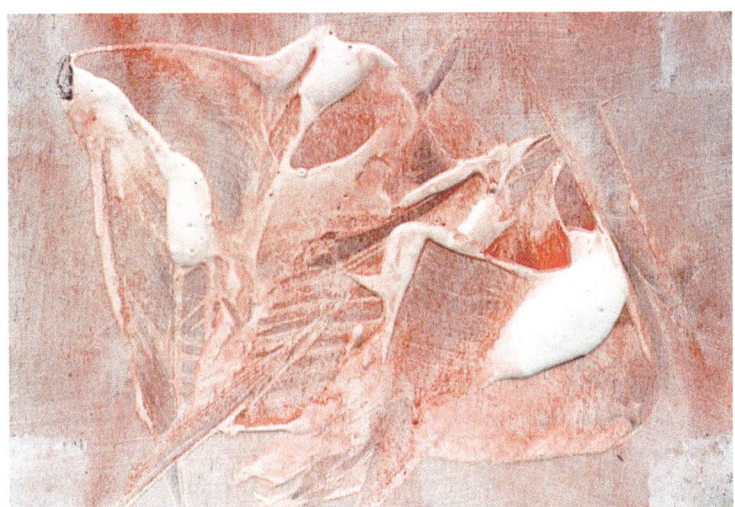

Spleen
Located near the liver and attached the stomach beneath the diaphragm,
the spleen is a body of lymphatic tissue active in the immune system of the body.

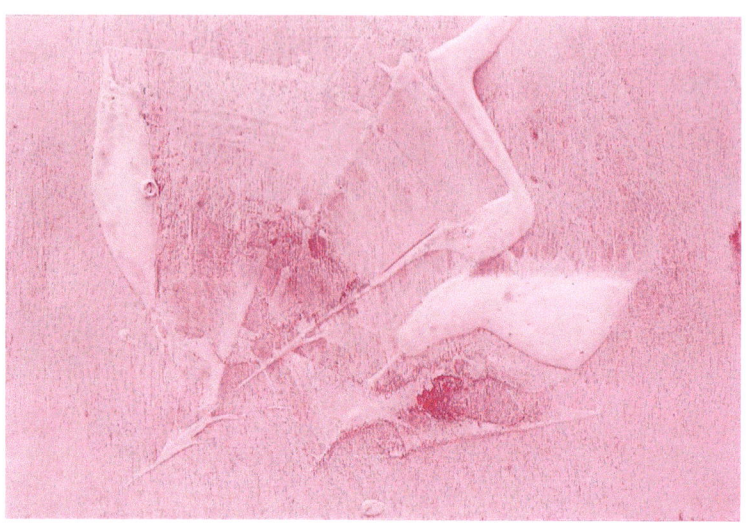

Stomach
Recepticle of ingested material, the stomach is a sac situated below the diaphragm.
Food enters from the esophagus via the cardiac sphincter, and exits at the lower end
from the duodenum via the pyloric sphincter. The stomach lining is composed of layers of
smooth muscle and flexible fibre.

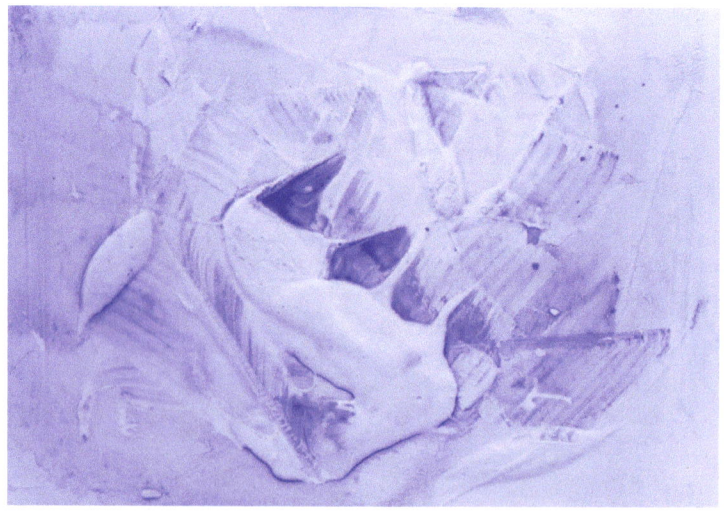

Teeth

The primary agents for biting, crushing and chewing food before swallowing and digestion. Thirty two permanent (adult) teeth are set in the upper and lower jaw. They are of varied size, shape and strength, and are used for different aspects of mastication.

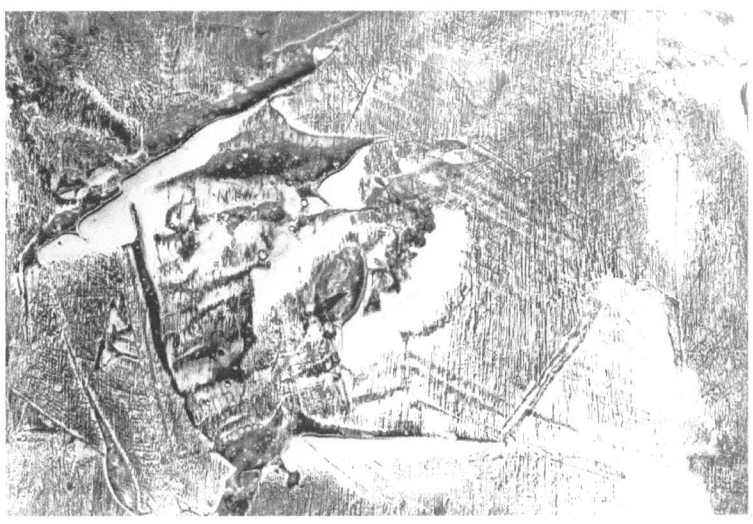

Testicles

A pair of sacs which form part of the male reproductive organ (penis), testicles contain testes where sperm cells are formed. The epidymis which encloses the testes stores the mature semen in tightly coiled tubes.

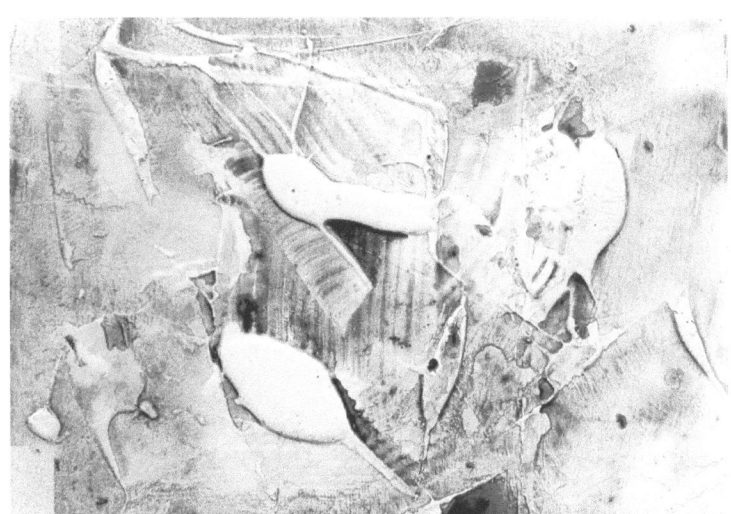

Thorax

The bones and muscles of the thorax protect and support the cavity of the ribcage. They act to support the spine, and movement of the head.

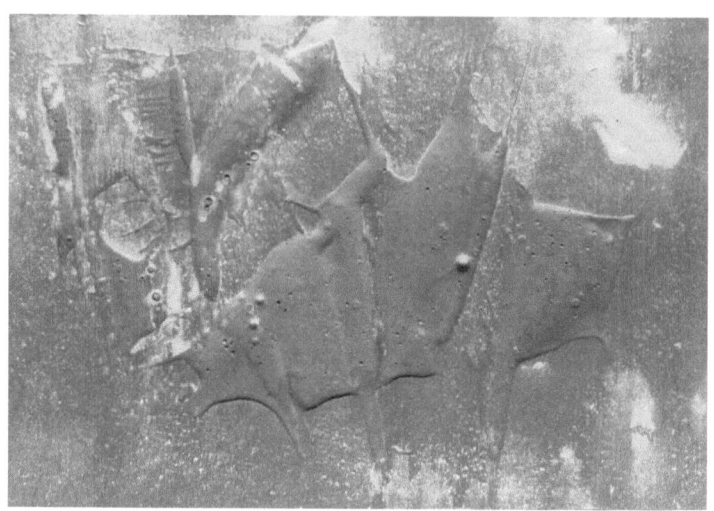

Thumb

Joined to the trapezium bone 0f the wrist the thumb is composed of three digits: the proximal, middle and distal phalanx. It operates in concert with the four fingers of the hand in gripping and holding actions.

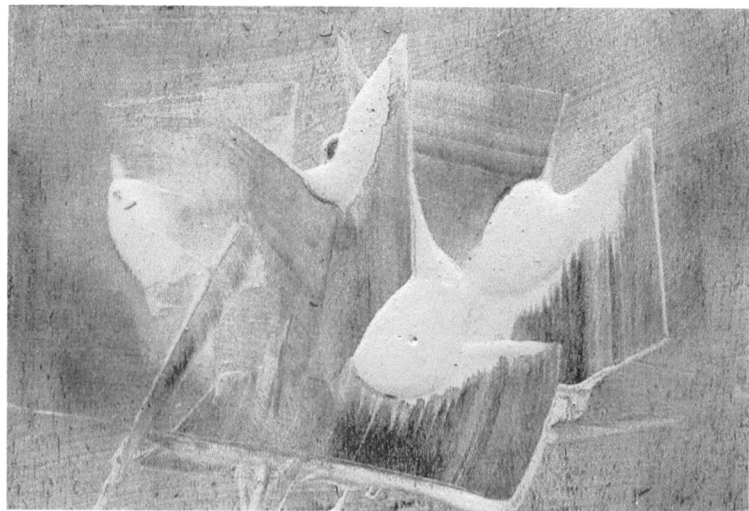

Throat
Pre-digested food and liquid passes from the oral cavity of the mouth
by muscular movement into the throat (pharynx) and then via the esophagus

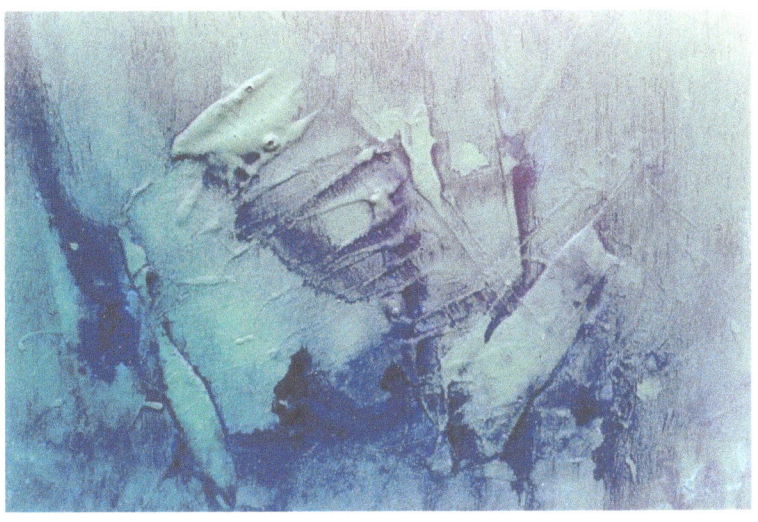

Tongue
The tongue, agent of taste and mastication, and in the shaping of articulated sound, lies in the cavity of the mouth. It is governed in its protruding movements by thegenioglossus and the styloglossus muscles, and is retracted by the hioglossus and elevated by the palatoglossus.

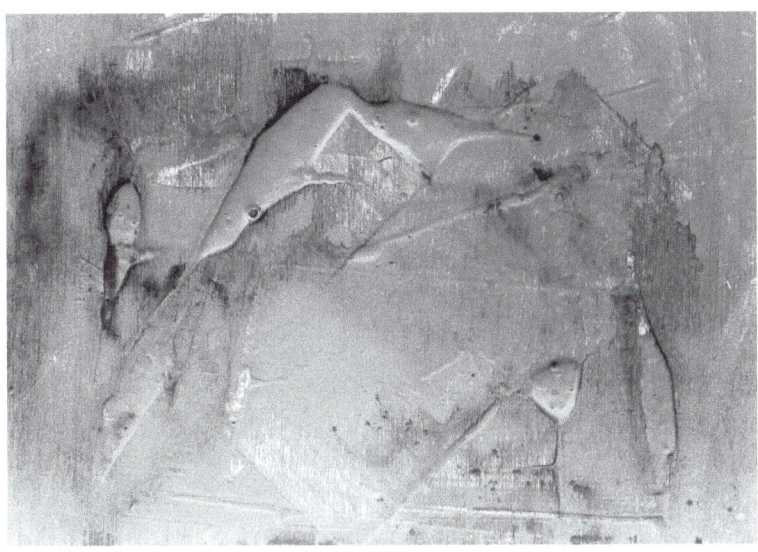

Veins
Vehicles for the transport of used blood vessels returned to the heart for re-circulation by a network of arteries.

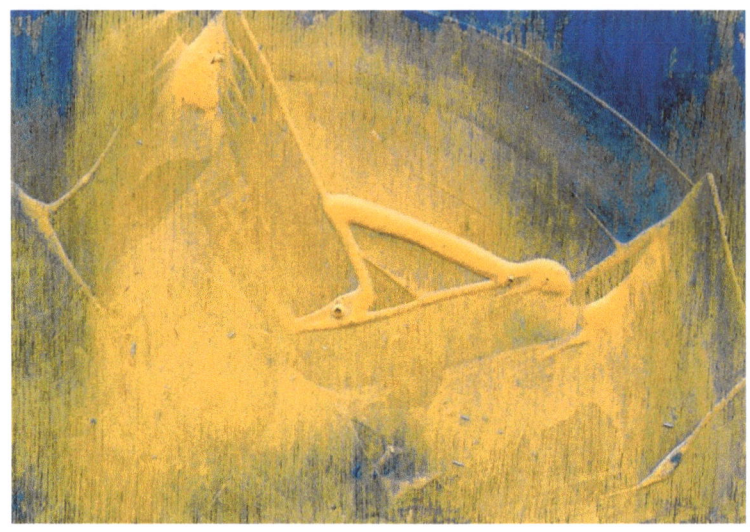

Wrist
At the extent of the lower arm the bones of the radius and ulna join with the hand at the prominent head of the wrist. The triquetal, pisiform and scaphoid bones provide a flexible junction for flexion of the complex of finger bones (phalanges).

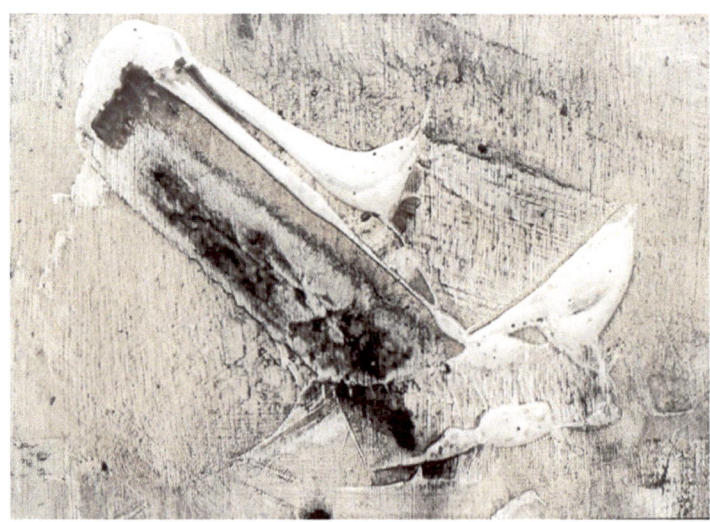

Anatomy Studies 2013

Emulsion on panel 16 x 12″

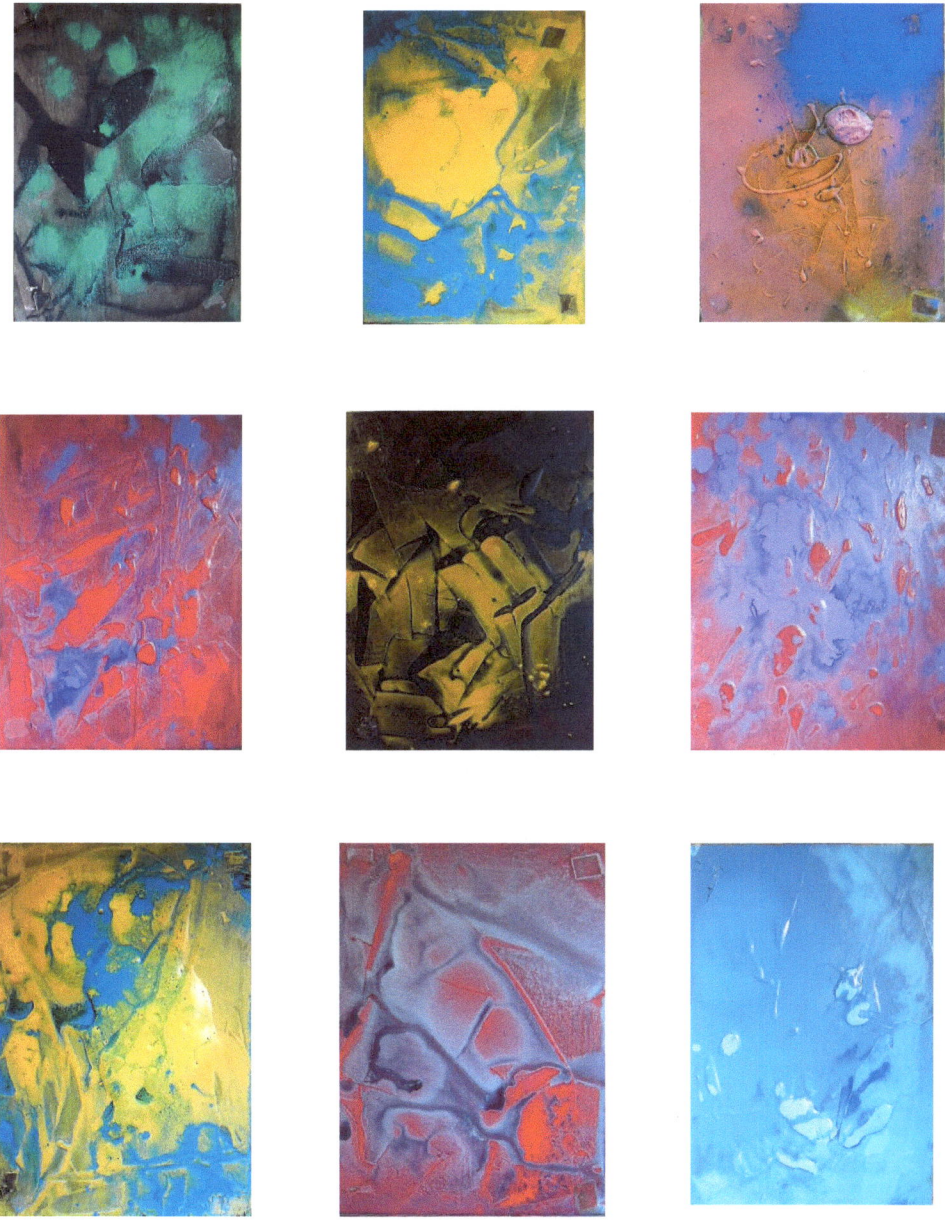

Axons

The long threadlike extension of a nerve cell that conducts nerve impulses from the cell body. The long portion of a neuron that conducts impulses away from the body of the cell. Also called nerve fibres.

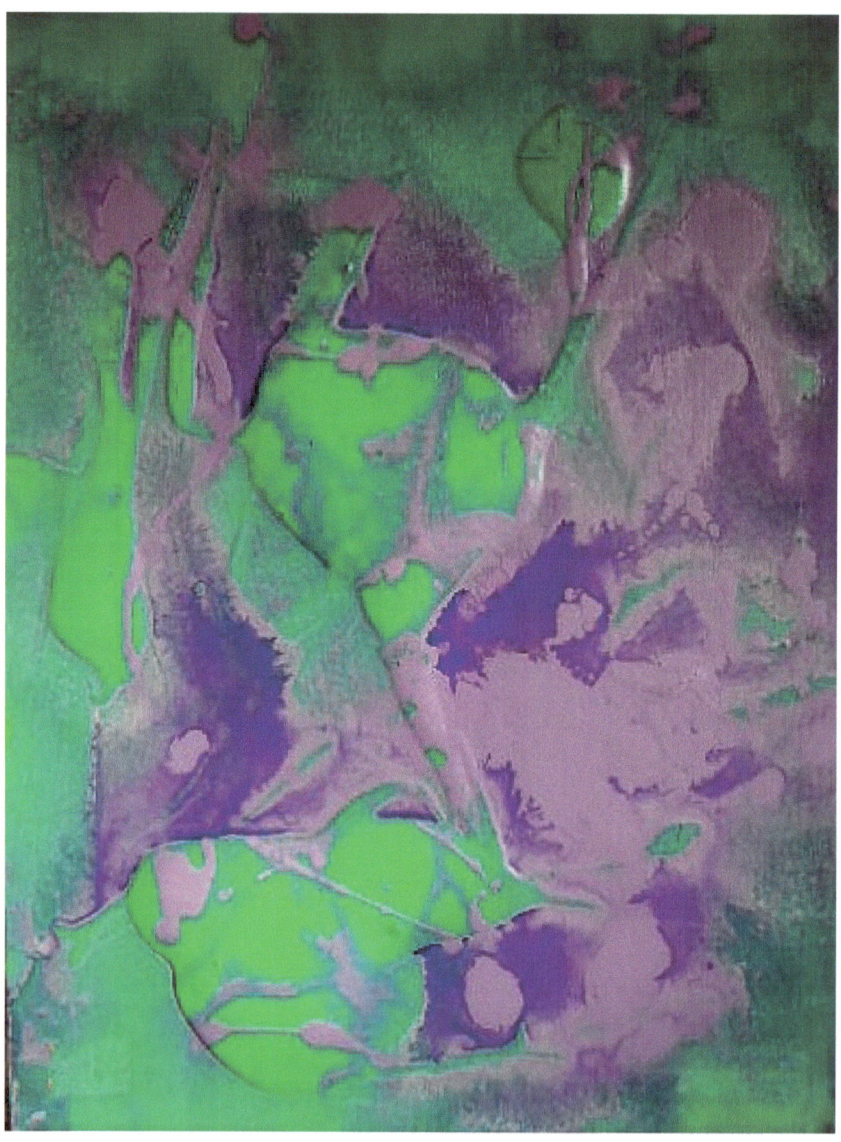

Bile Duct

Large and complicated reddish-brown glandular organ located in the upper right portion of the abdominal cavity; secretes bile and functions in metabolism of protein and carbohydrate and fat; synthesizes substances involved in the clotting of the blood; synthesizes vitamin A; detoxifies poisonous substances and breaks down worn-out erythrocytesThe excretory passages in the liver that carry bile to the hepatic duct, which joins with the cystic duct to form the common bile duct opening into the duodenum.

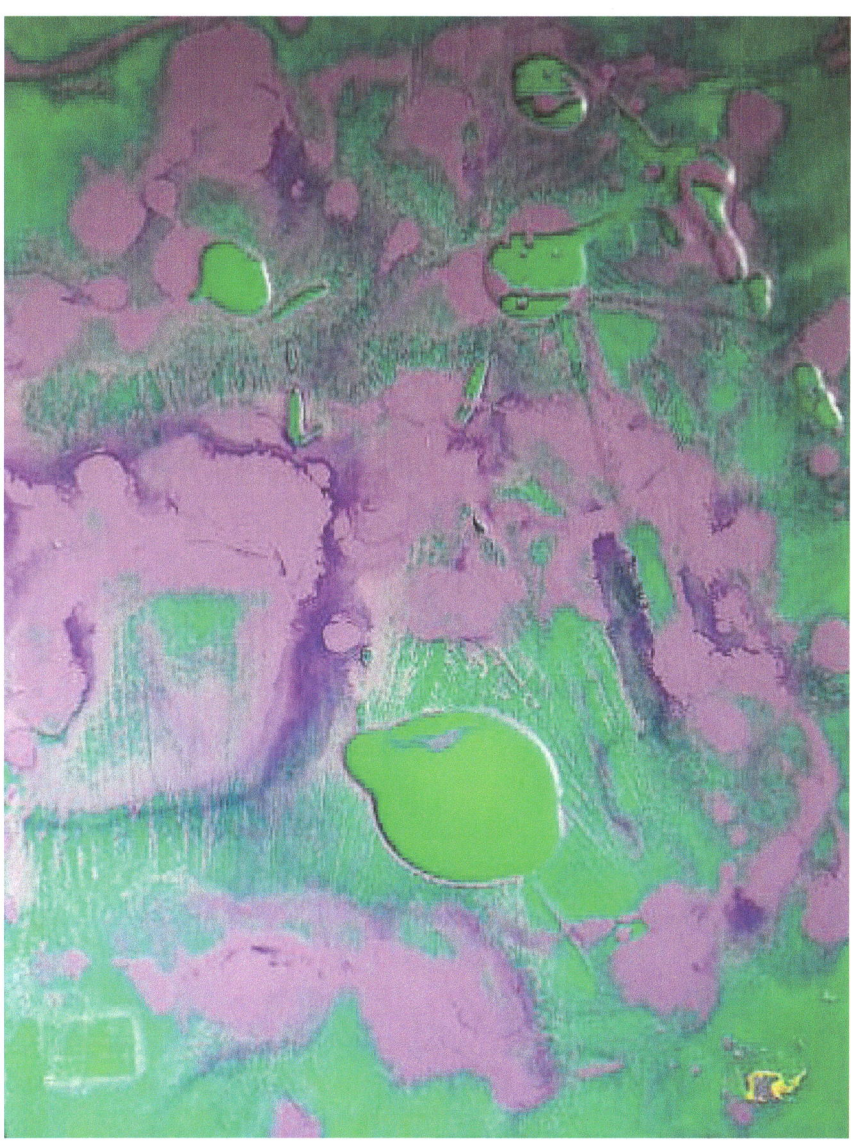

Bone Marrow

The soft, fatty, vascular tissue that fills most bone cavities and is the source of red blood cells and many white blood cells. The spongy, red tissue that fills the bone cavities of mammals. Bone marrow is the source of red blood cells, platelets, and most white blood cells

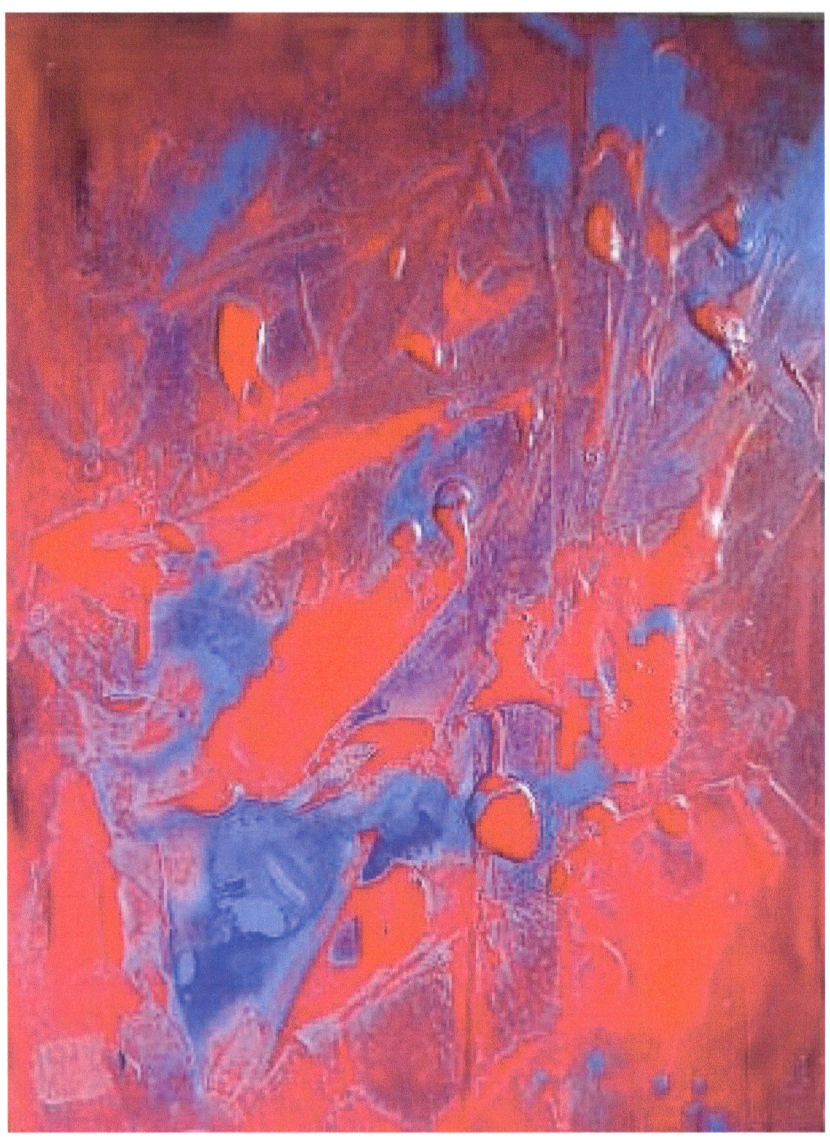

Deltoids

A thick triangular muscle covering the shoulder joint, used to raise the arm from the side. The gluteal muscles, the quadriceps, calves, anterior **deltoids** of the shoulders, and erector spinae are the most important drive phase muscles for acceleration.

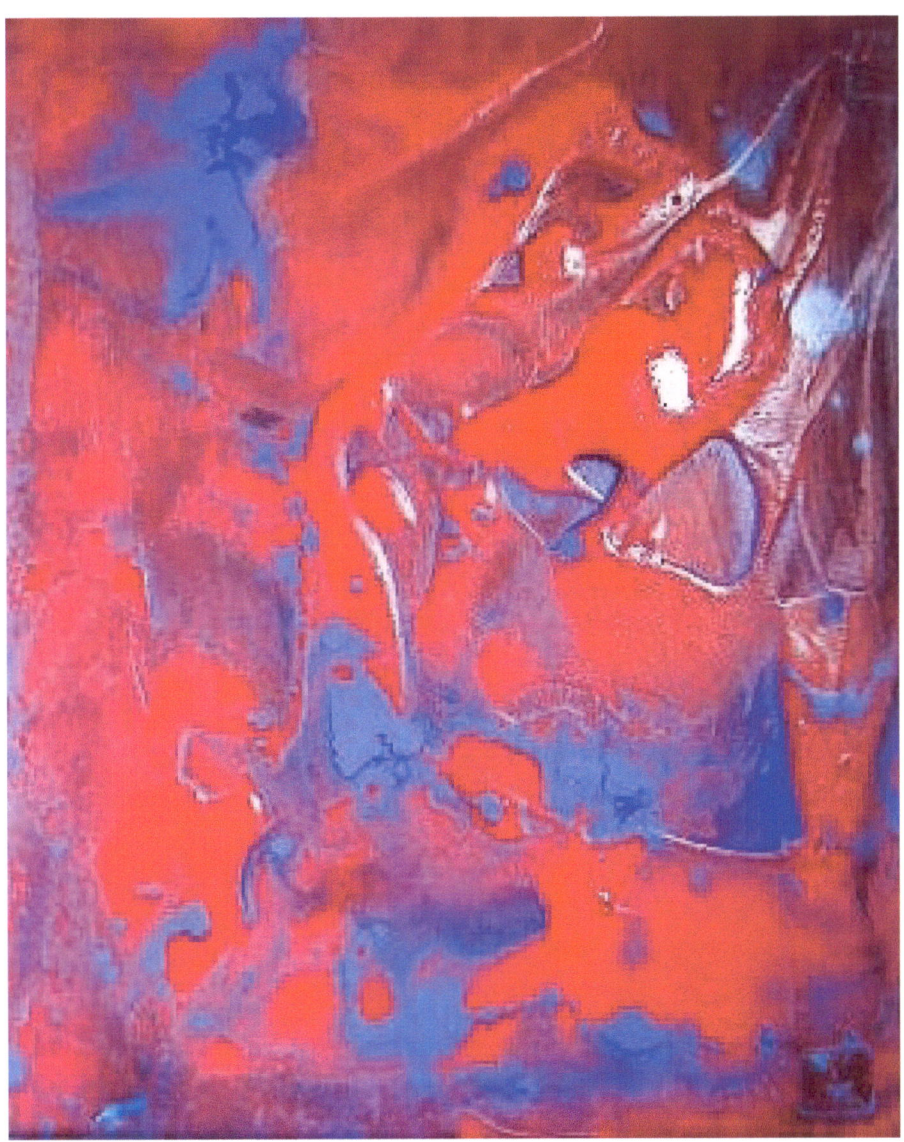

Diaphragm

The large muscle that separates the chest cavity from the abdominal cavity in mammals and is the principal muscle of respiration. As the diaphragm contracts and moves downward, the lungs expand and air moves into them. As the diaphragm relaxes and moves upward, the lungs contract and air is forced out of them.

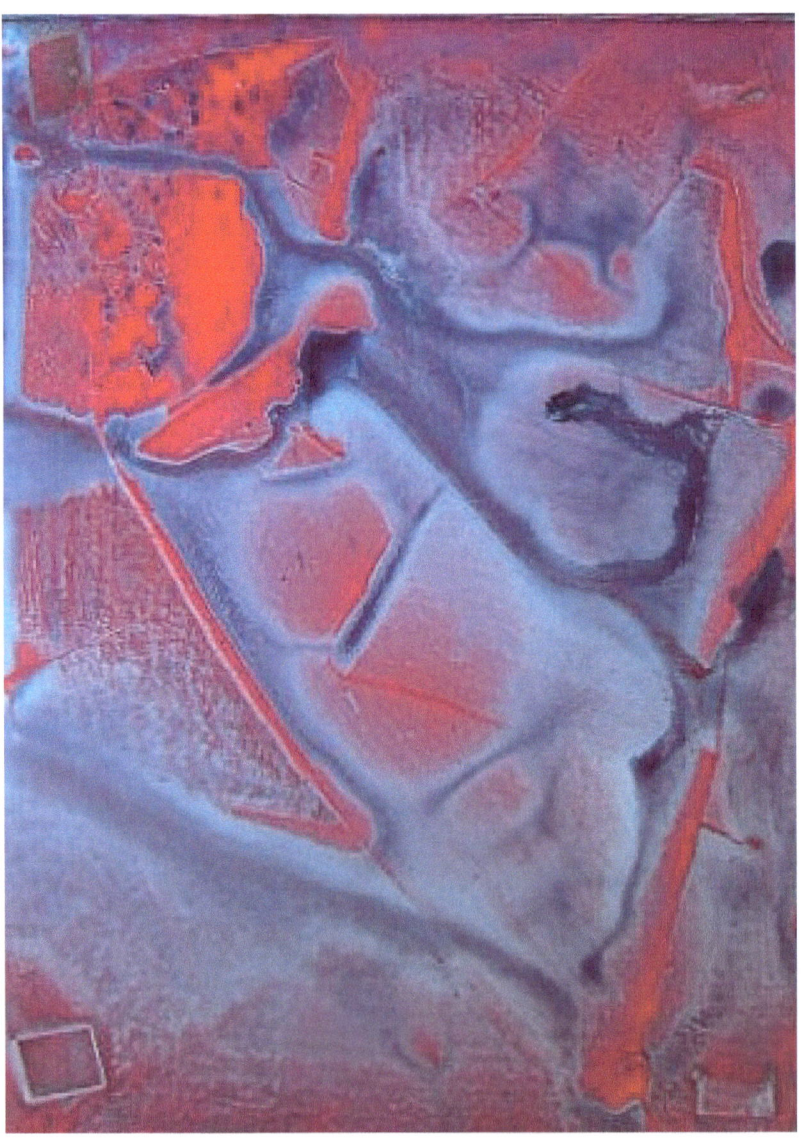

Epidermis

The protective outer layer of the skin. In invertebrate animals, the epidermis is made up of a single layer of cells. In vertebrates, it is made up of many layers of cells and overlies the dermis. Hair and feathers grow from the epidermis

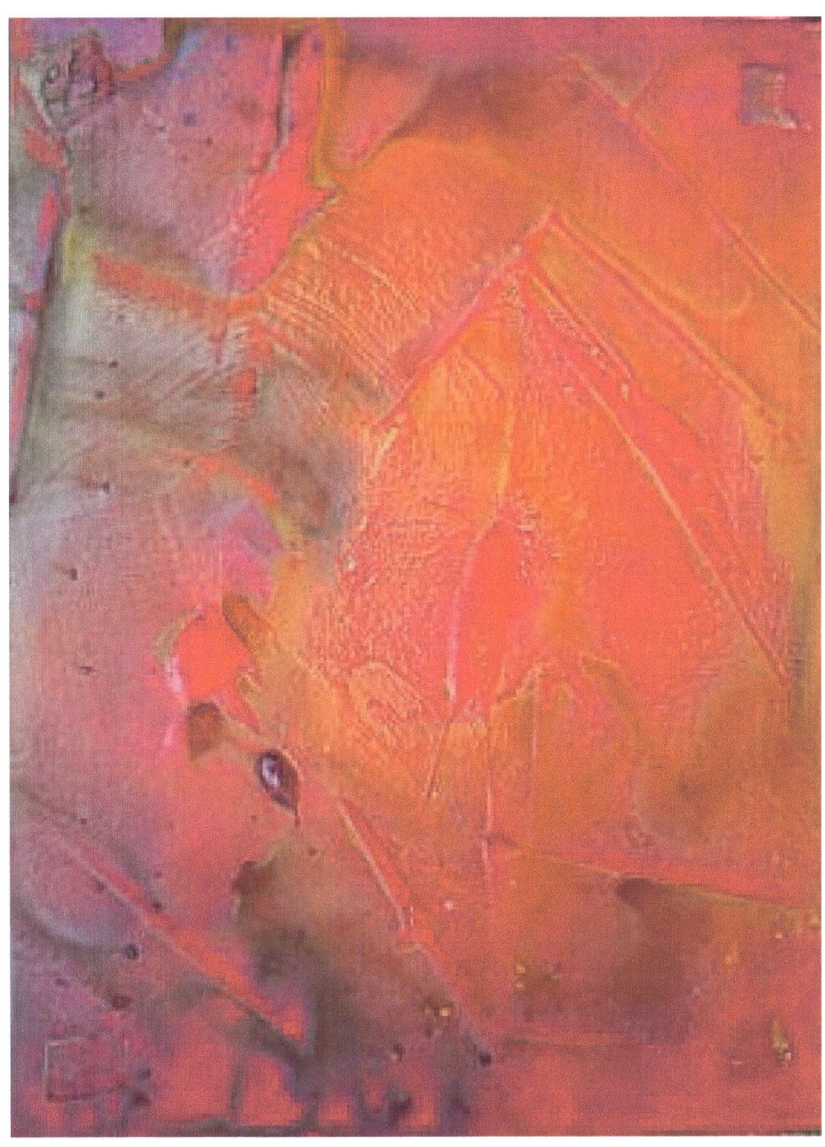

Fibre

A narrow elongated thick-walled cell: a constituent of sclerenchyma tissue. The basic structural and functional unit of all organisms; they may exist as independent units of life (as in monads) or may form colonies or tissues as in higher plants and animals

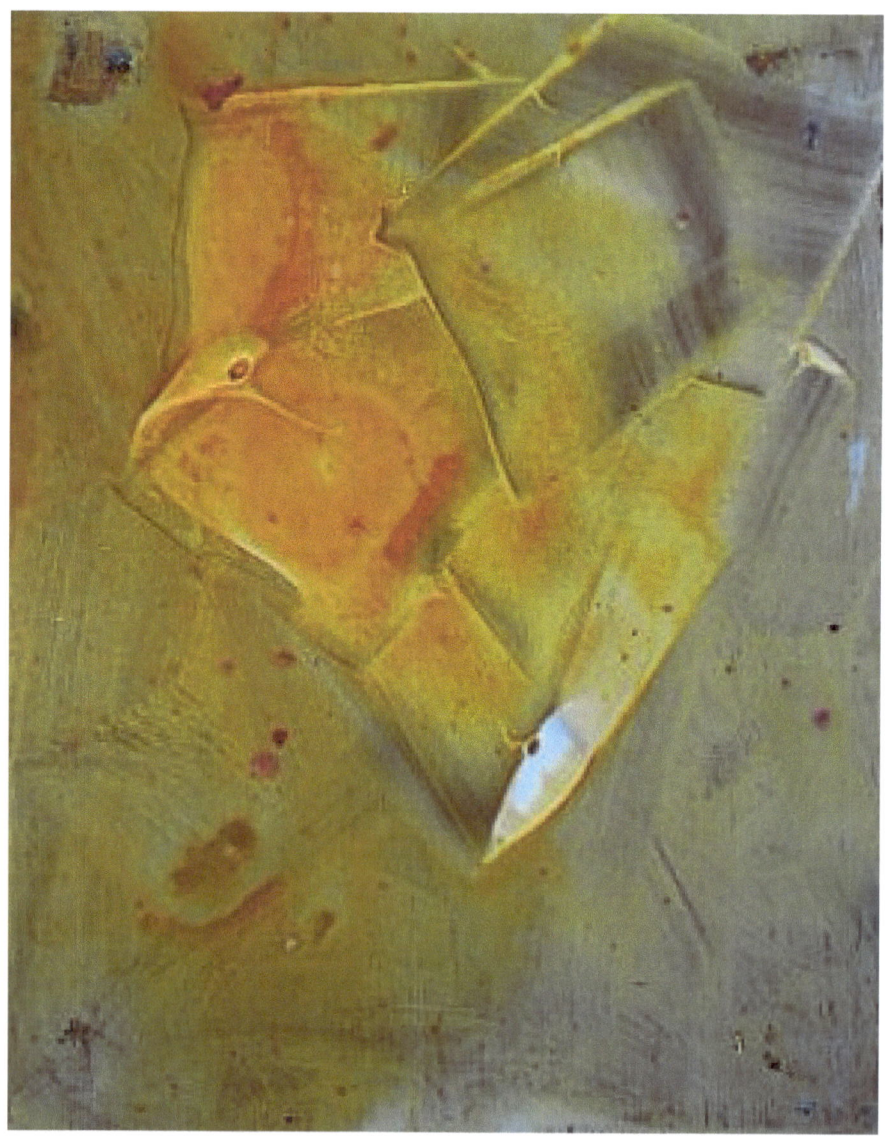

Filament
a threadlike structure (as a chainlike series of cells

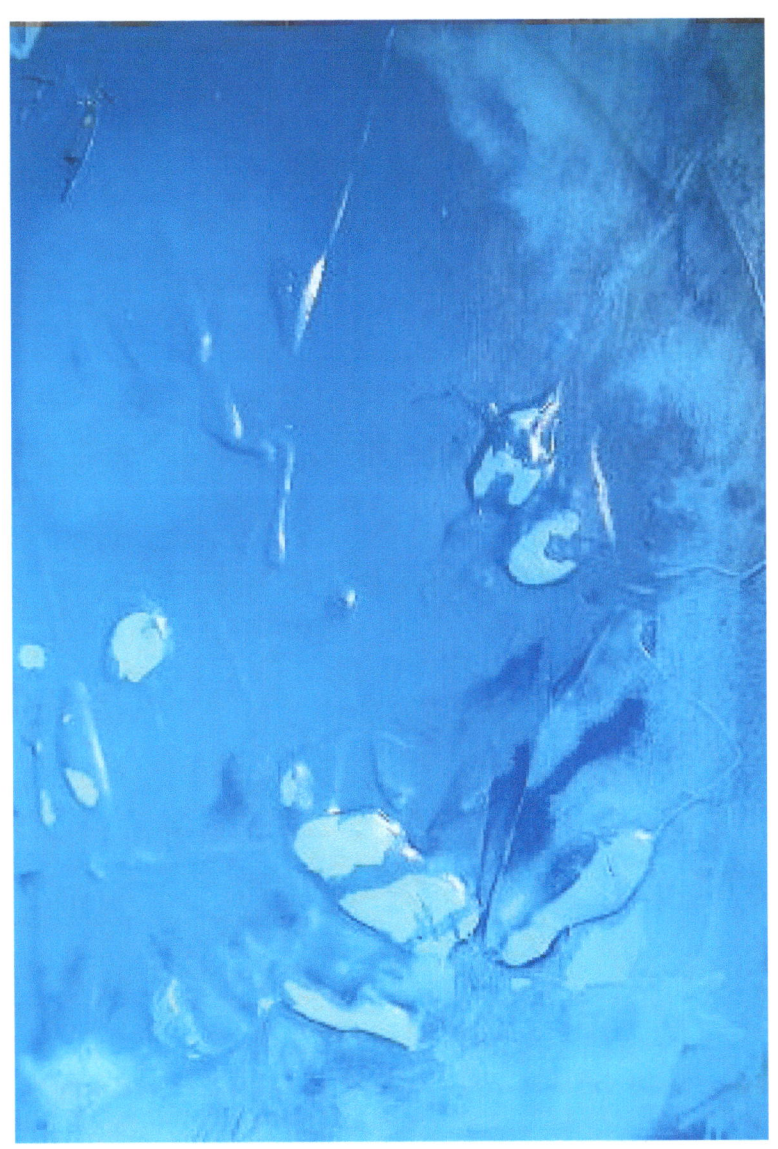

Gallbladder

A small, pear-shaped muscular sac in most vertebrates in which bile is stored. The gallbladder is located beneath the liver and secretes bile into the duodenum of the small intestine.

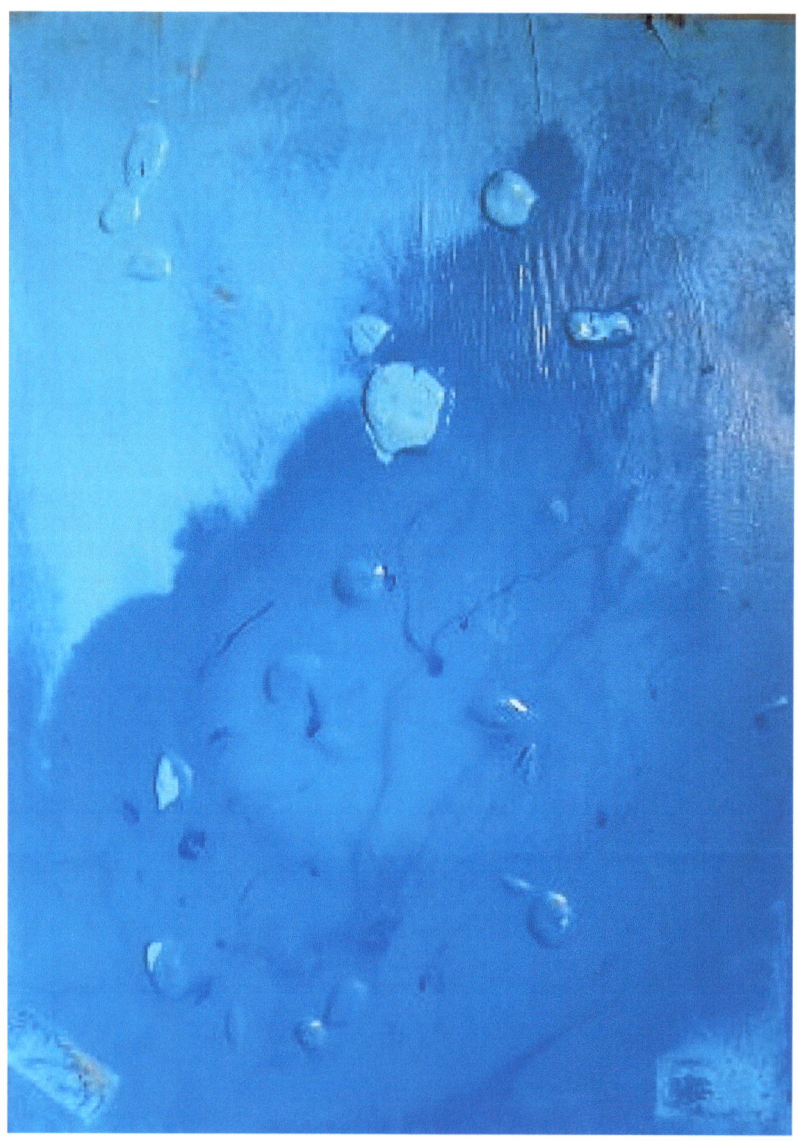

Humerus

A bump on the outside of the humerus where the deltoid muscle attaches. Technically the part of the superior limb between the shoulder and the elbow but commonly used to refer to the whole superior limb.

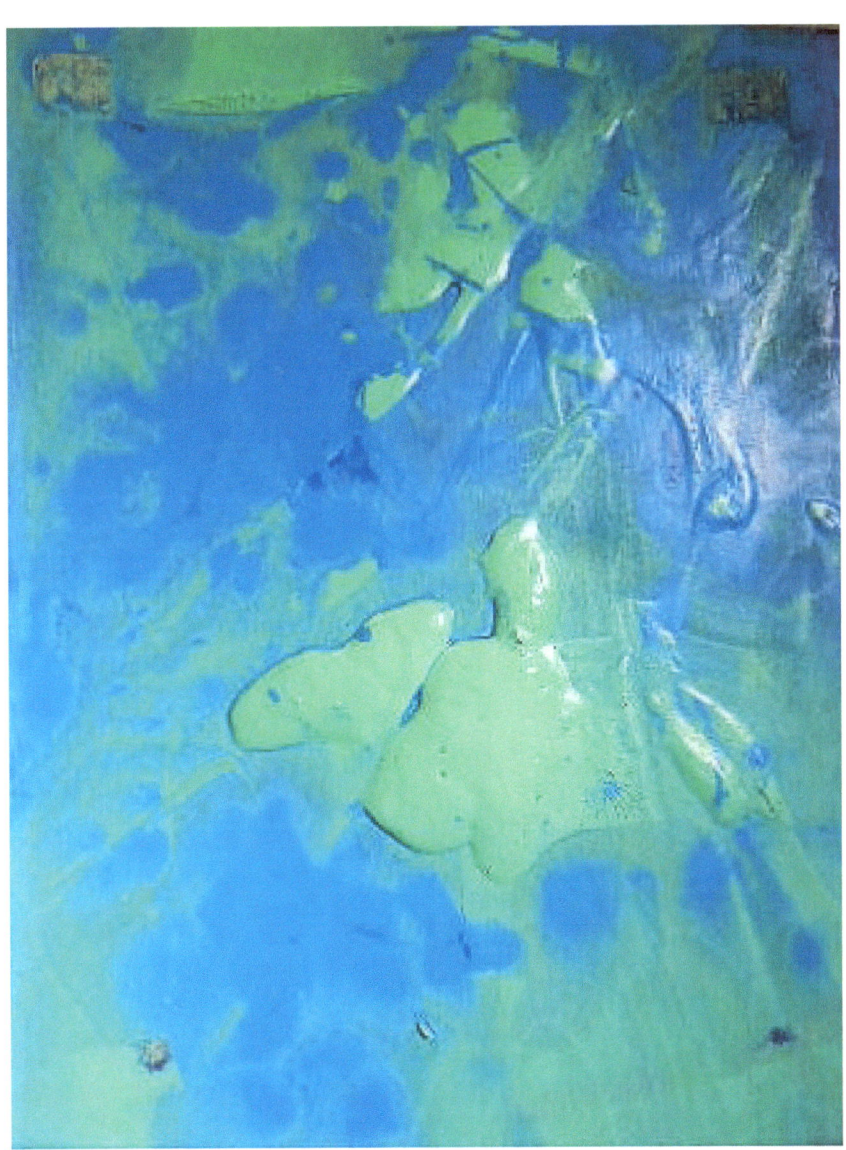

Intestine

The portion of the alimentary canal extending from the stomach to the anus and, in humans and other mammals, consisting of two segments, the small intestine and the large intestine. The muscular tube that forms the part of the digestive tract extending from the stomach to the anus and consisting of the small and large intestines. In the intestine, nutrients and water from digested food are absorbed and waste products are solidified into faeces.

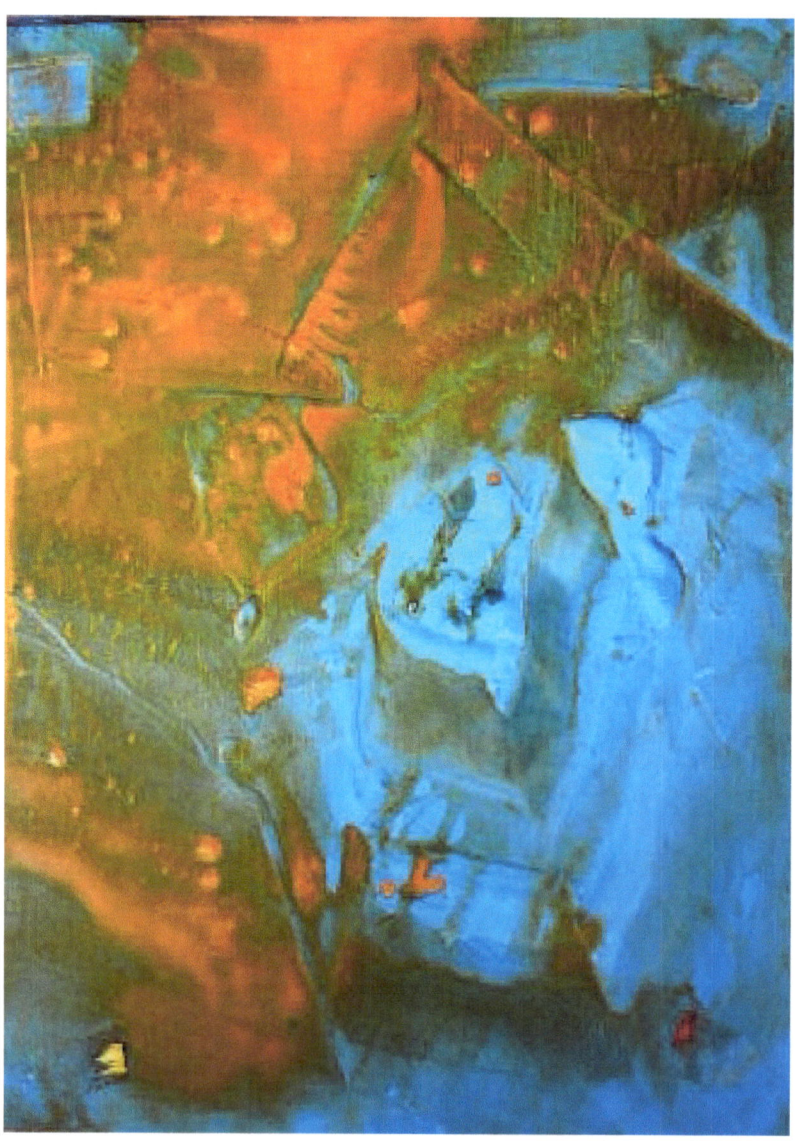

Ions

An atom or a group of atoms that has an electric charge. Positive ions, or cations, are formed by the loss of electrons; negative ions, or anions, are formed by the gain of electrons.

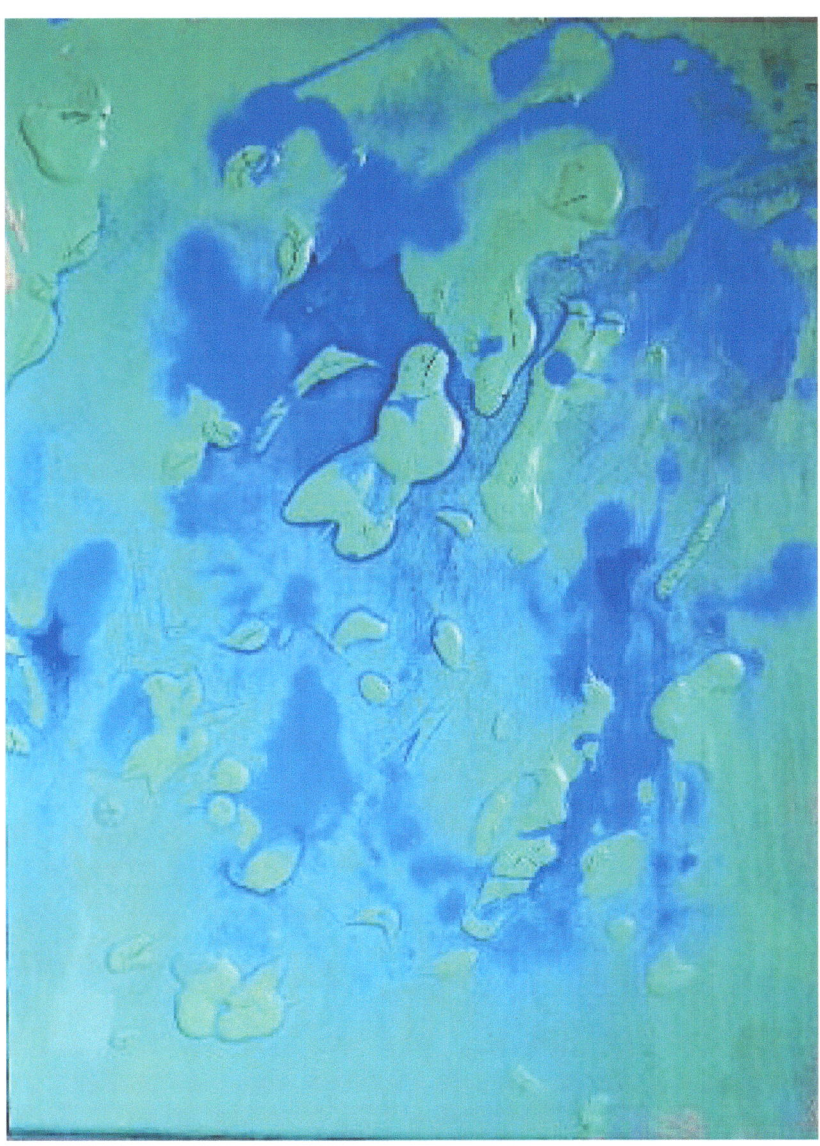

Kidney

A pair of organs that are located in the rear of the abdominal cavity in vertebrates. The kidneys regulate fluid balance in the body and filter out wastes from the blood in the form of urine. The functional unit of the kidney is the nephron. Wastes filtered from the blood by the nephrons drain into the ureters, muscular tubes that connect each kidney to the bladder.

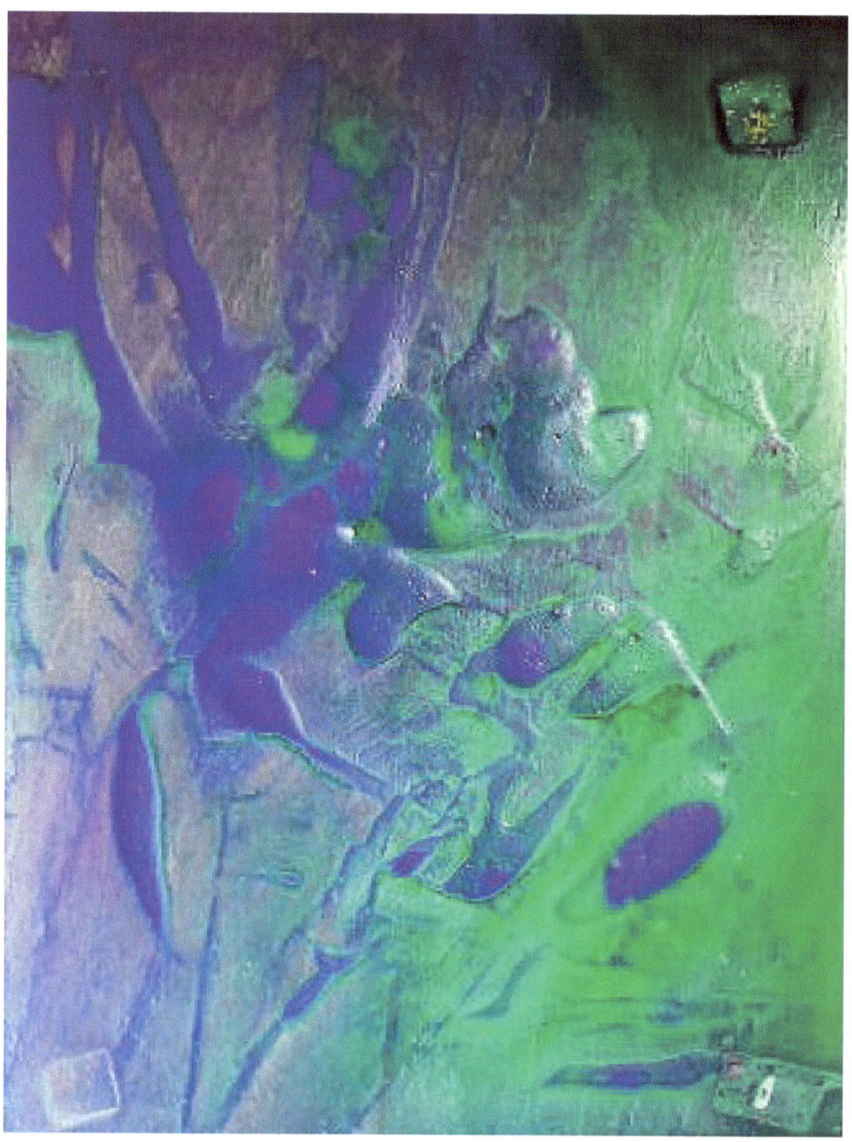

Lever

Any one of the numerous bones and associated joints of the body that act as a simple machine so that force applied to one end of the bone tends to rotate the bone in the direction opposite from that of the applied force.

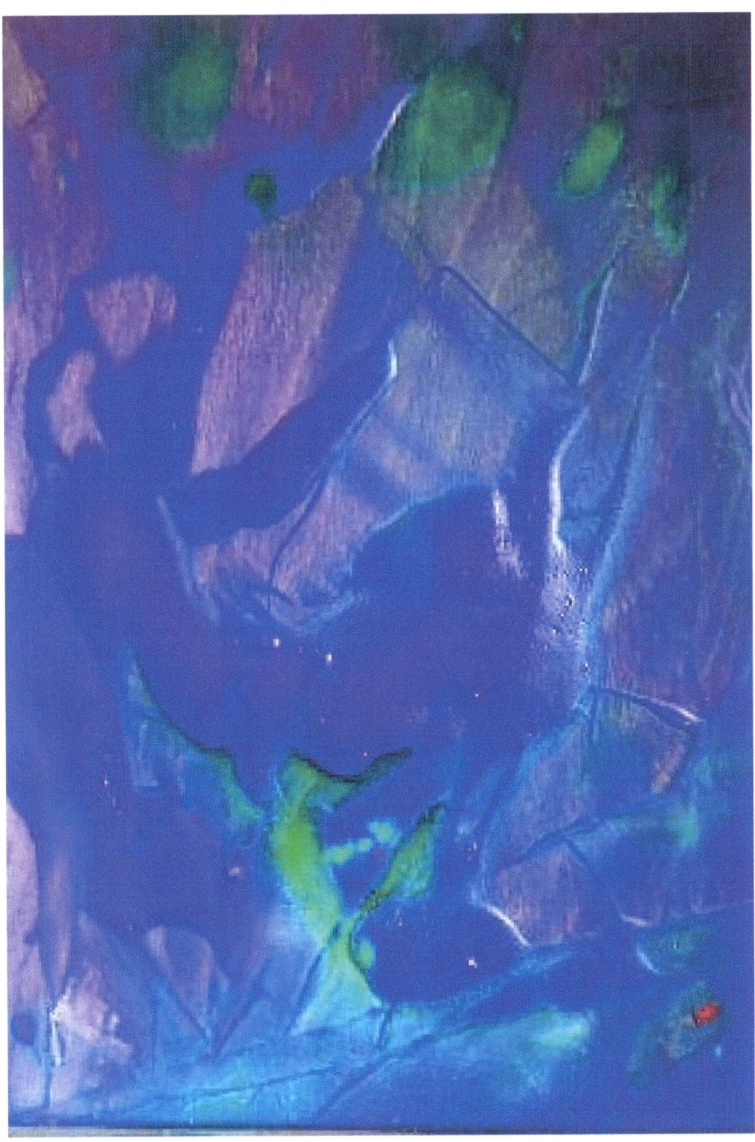

Liver

The largest gland of the body, lying beneath the diaphragm in the upper right portion of the abdominal cavity, which secretes bile and is active in the formation of certain blood proteins and in the metabolism of carbohydrates, fats, and proteins.

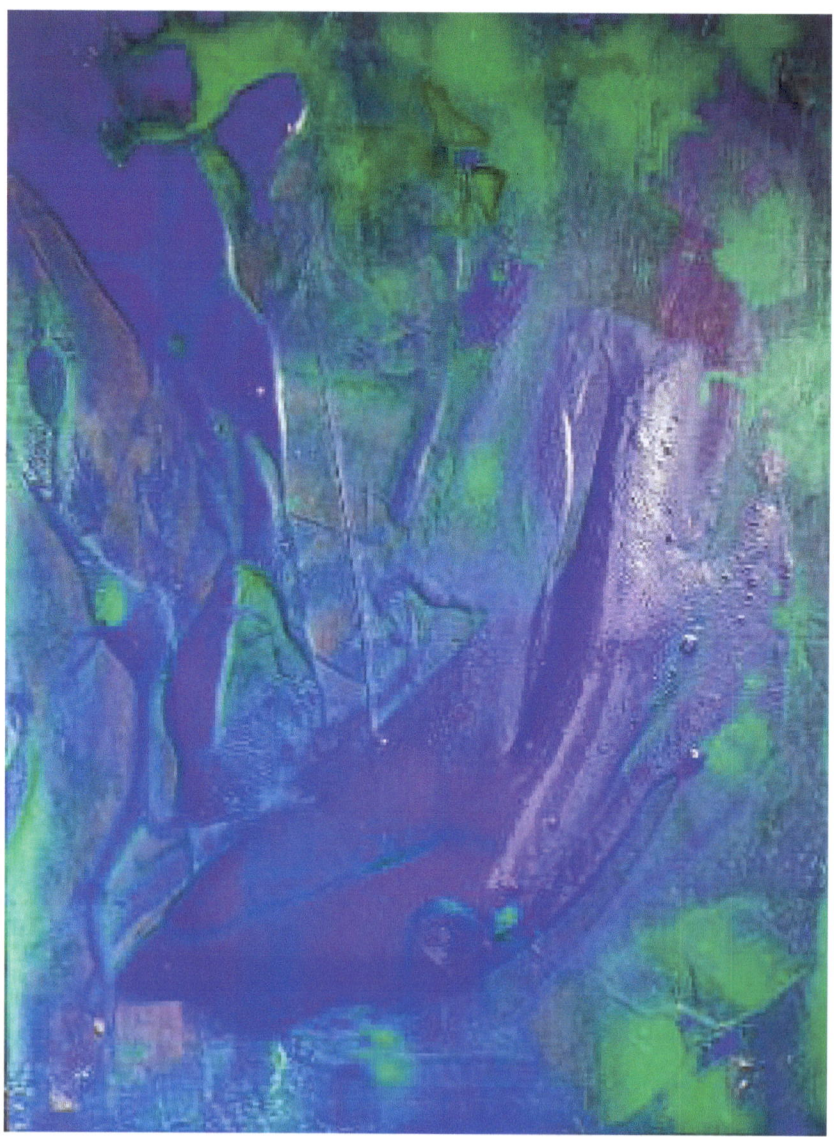

Lymph Nodes

Small, bean-shaped masses of tissue scattered along the lymphatic system that act as filters and immune monitors, removing fluids, bacteria, or cancer cells that travel through the lymph system. Breast cancer cells in the lymph nodes under the arm or in the chest are a sign that the cancer has spread, and that it might recur.

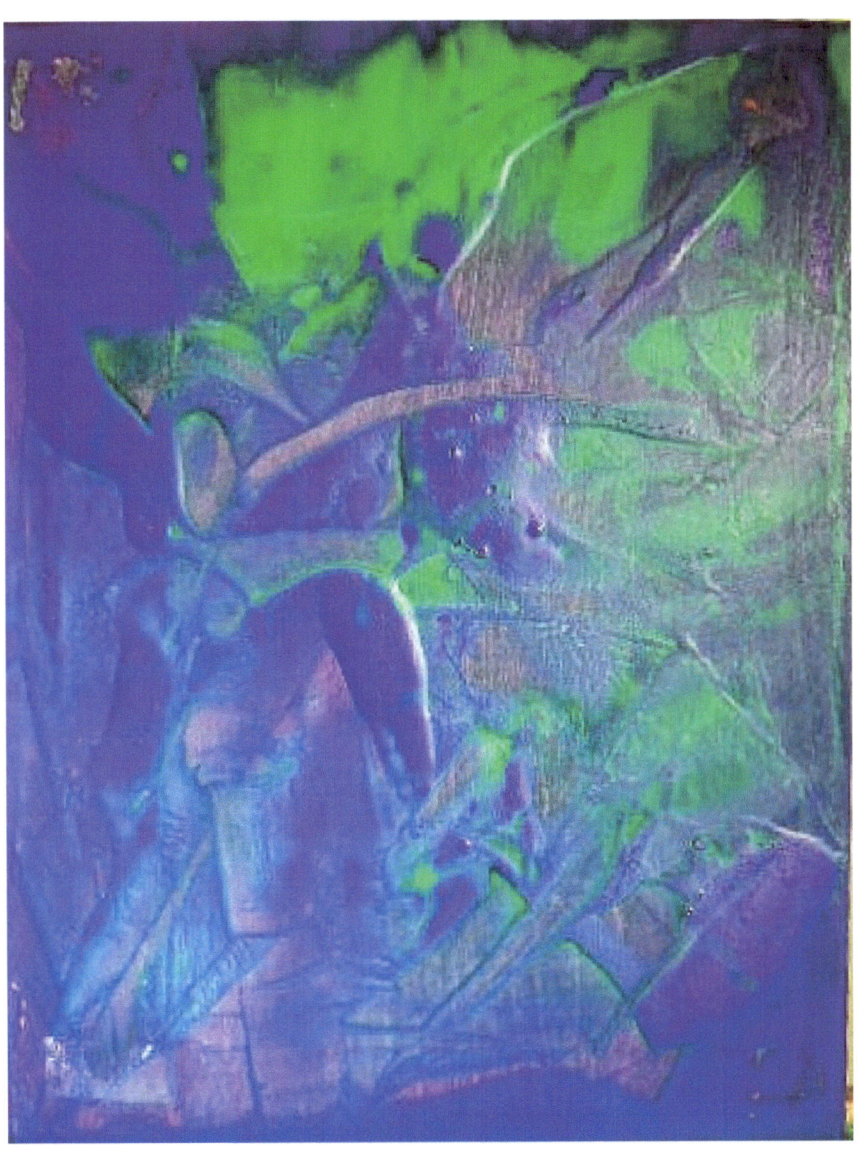

Meninges

A series of membranous layers of connective tissue that protect the central nervous system (brain and spinal cord). Damage or infection to the meninges, such as in meningitis, can cause serious neurological damage and even death.

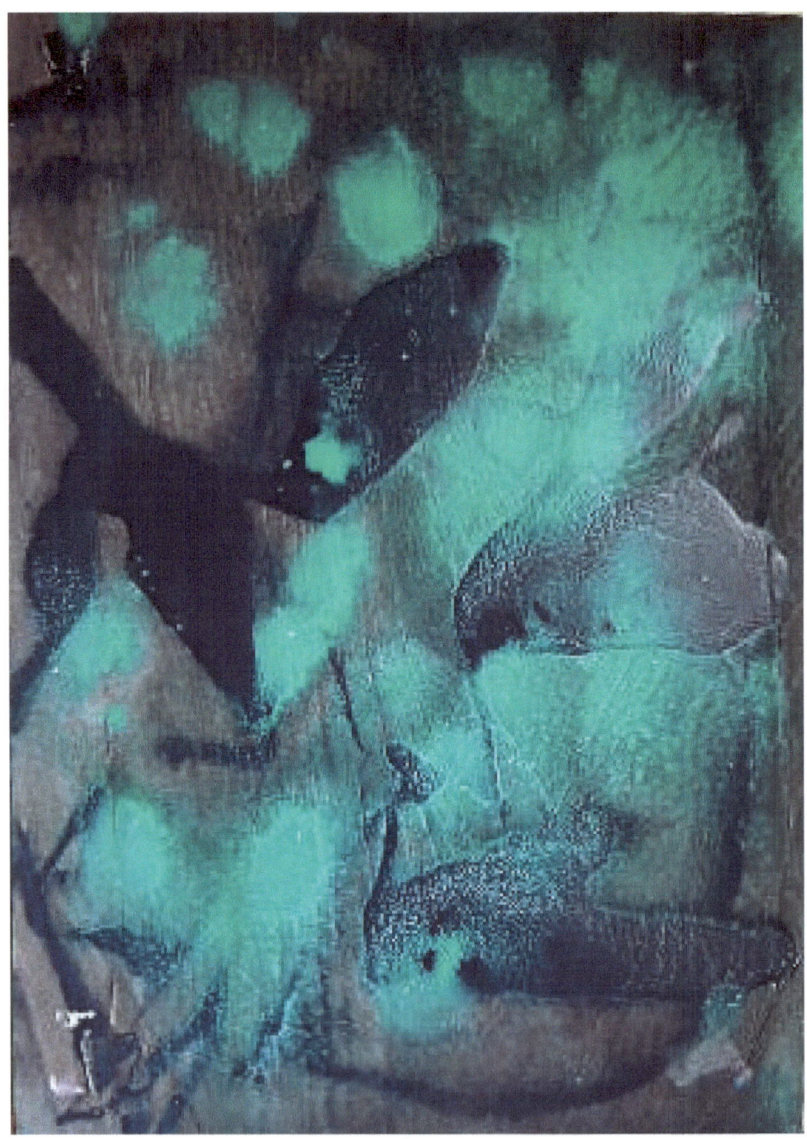

Molecules

A unit of matter that is the smallest particle of an element or chemical combination of atoms (as a compound) capable of retaining chemical identity with the substance in mass.

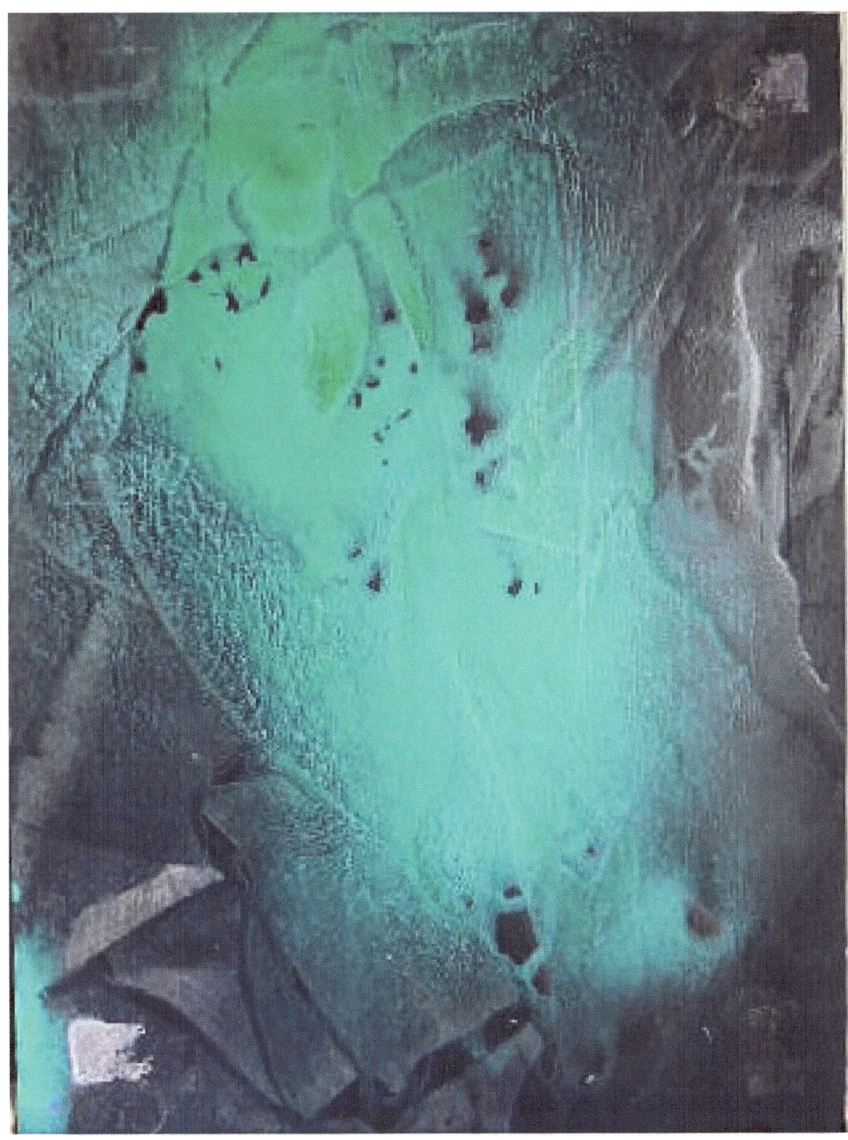

Monocytes

The largest of the white blood cells. They have one nucleus and a large amount of grayish-blue cytoplasm. Develop into macrophages and both consume foreign material and alert T cells to its presence

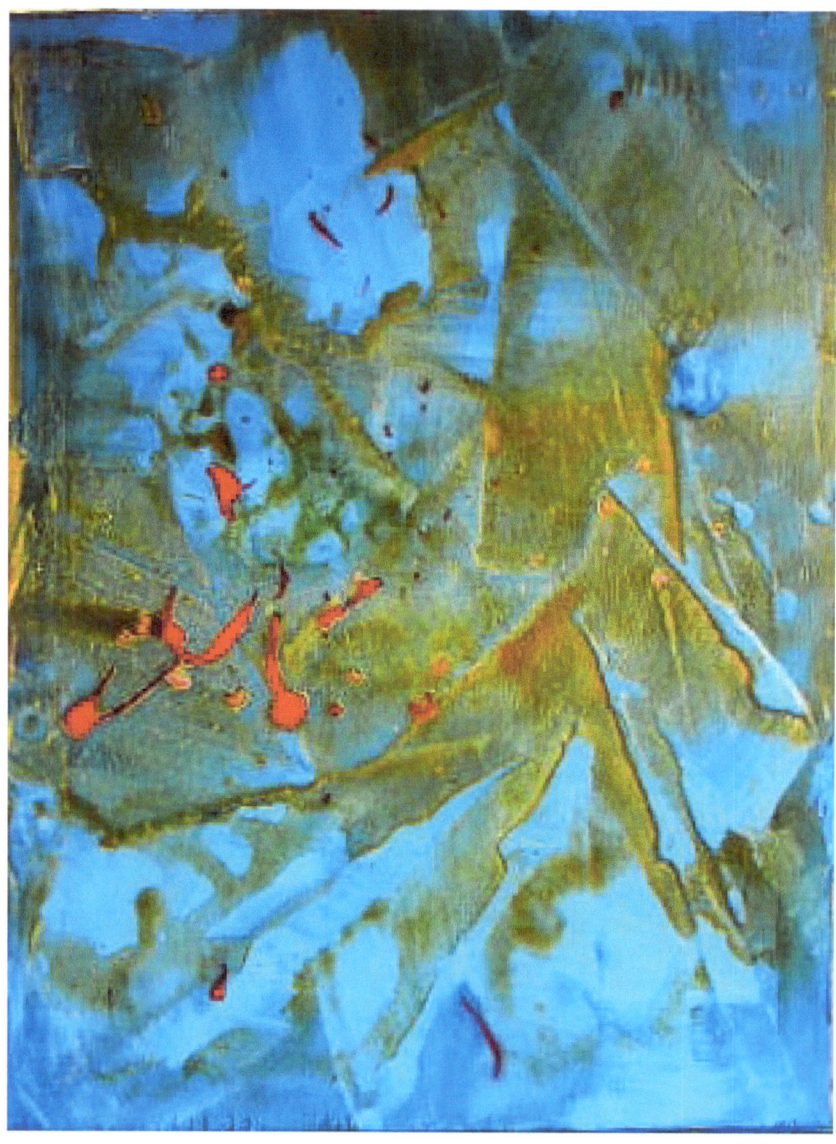

Motor
A muscle, nerve, or center that effects movements.

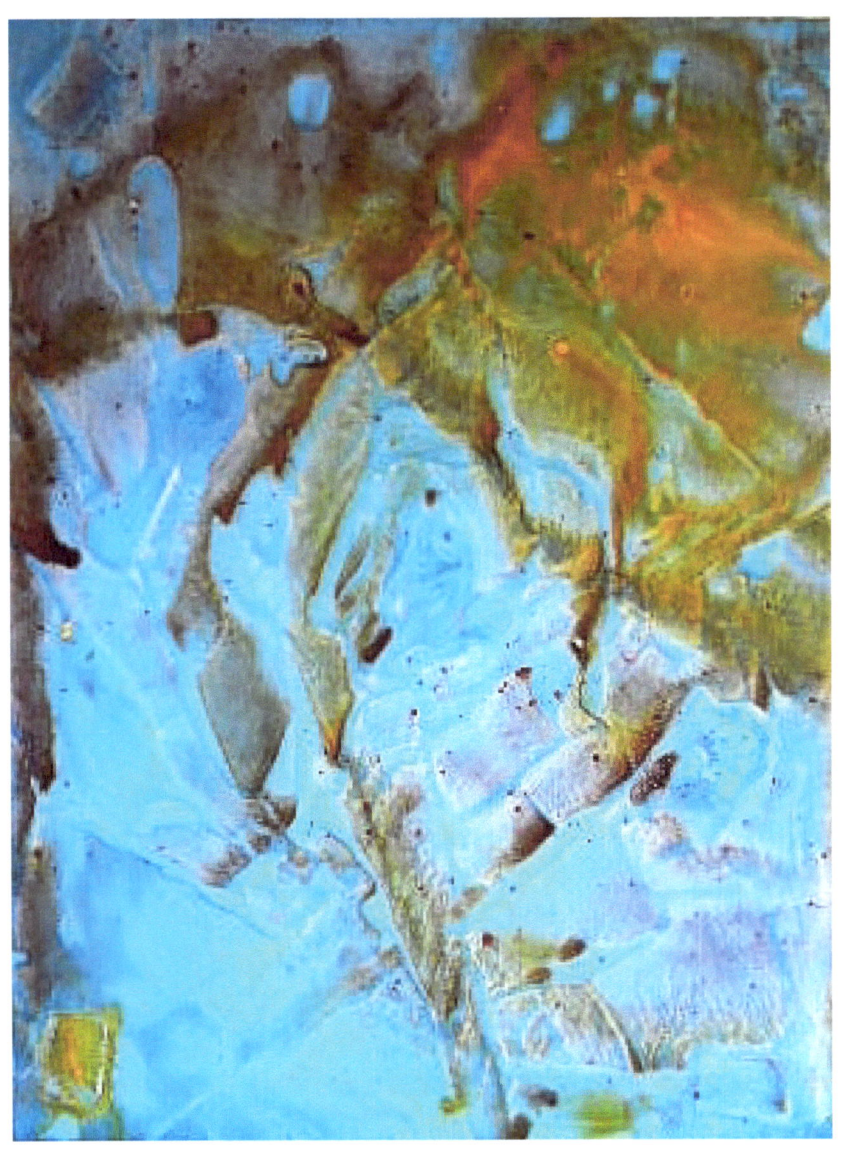

Mucus

The free slime of the mucous membrane, composed of the secretion of its glands, various salts, desquamated cells and leukocytes.

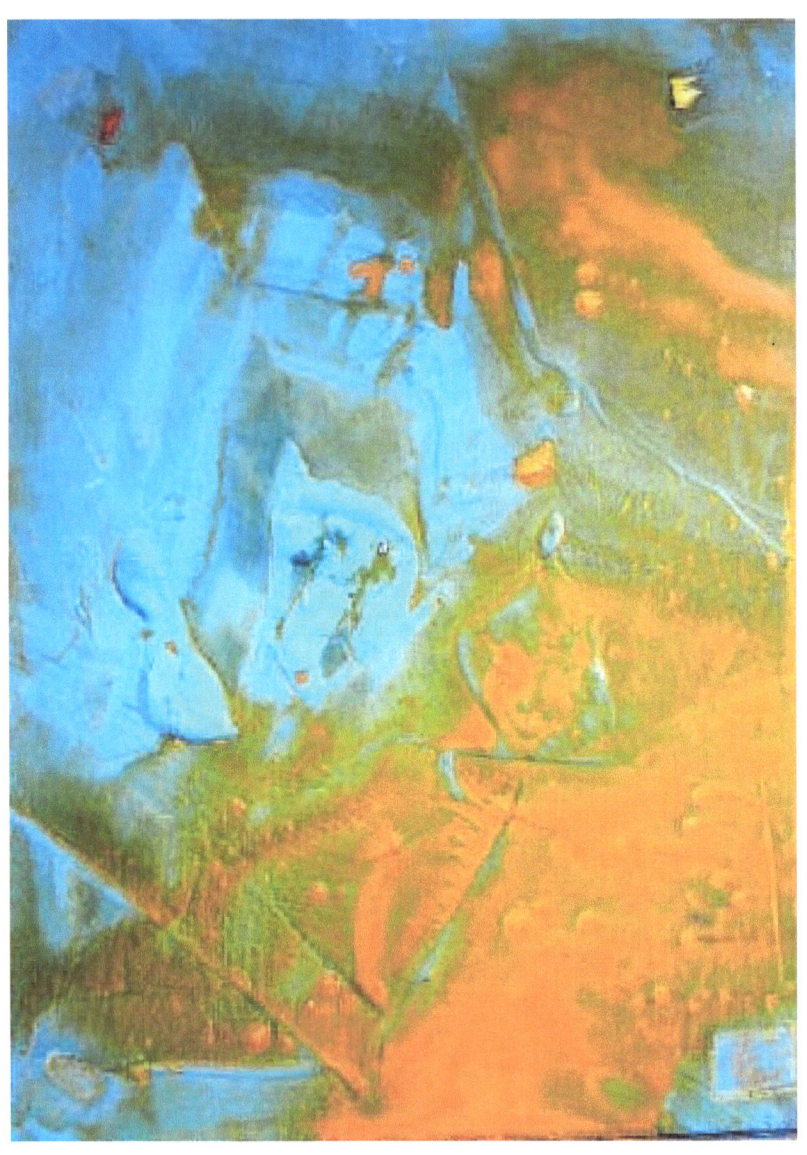

Nails
The horny cutaneous plate on the dorsal surface of the distal end of a finger or toe.

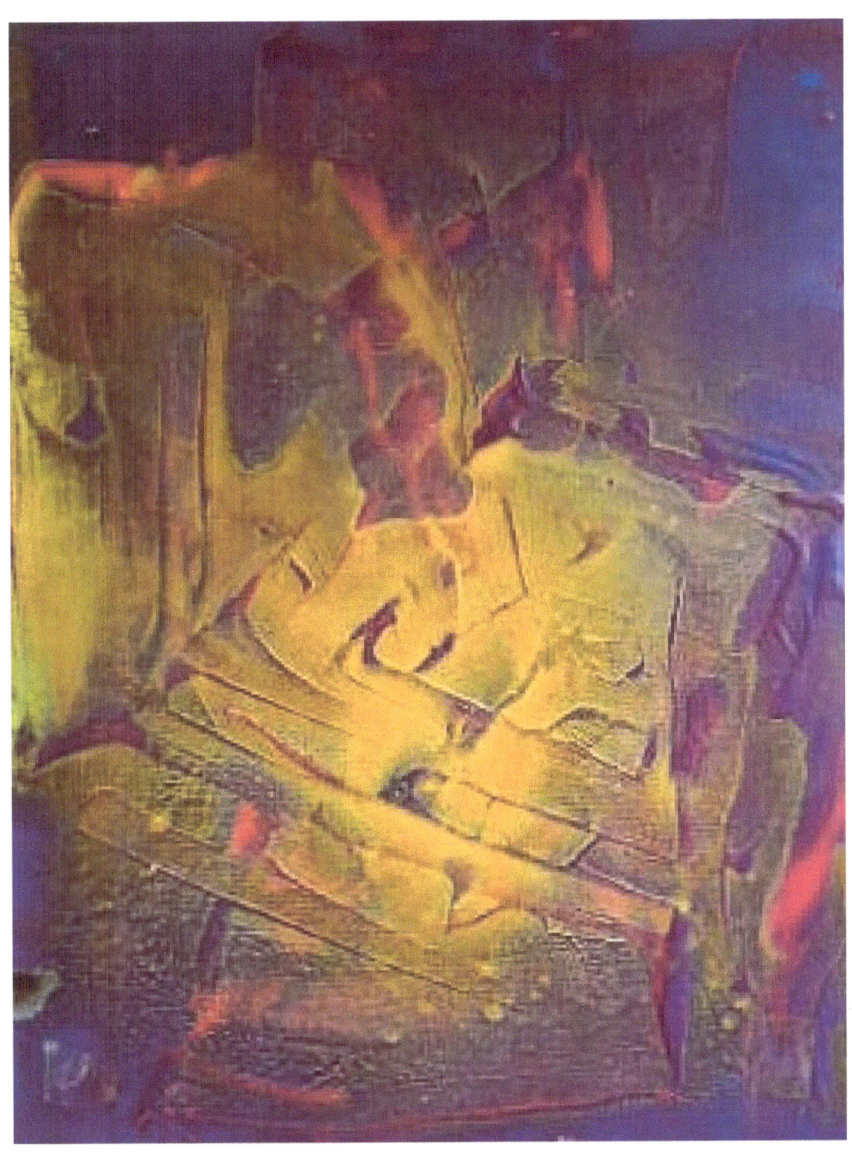

Neurons
Nerve cells in the brain, brain stem, and spinal cord that connect the nervous system and the muscles.

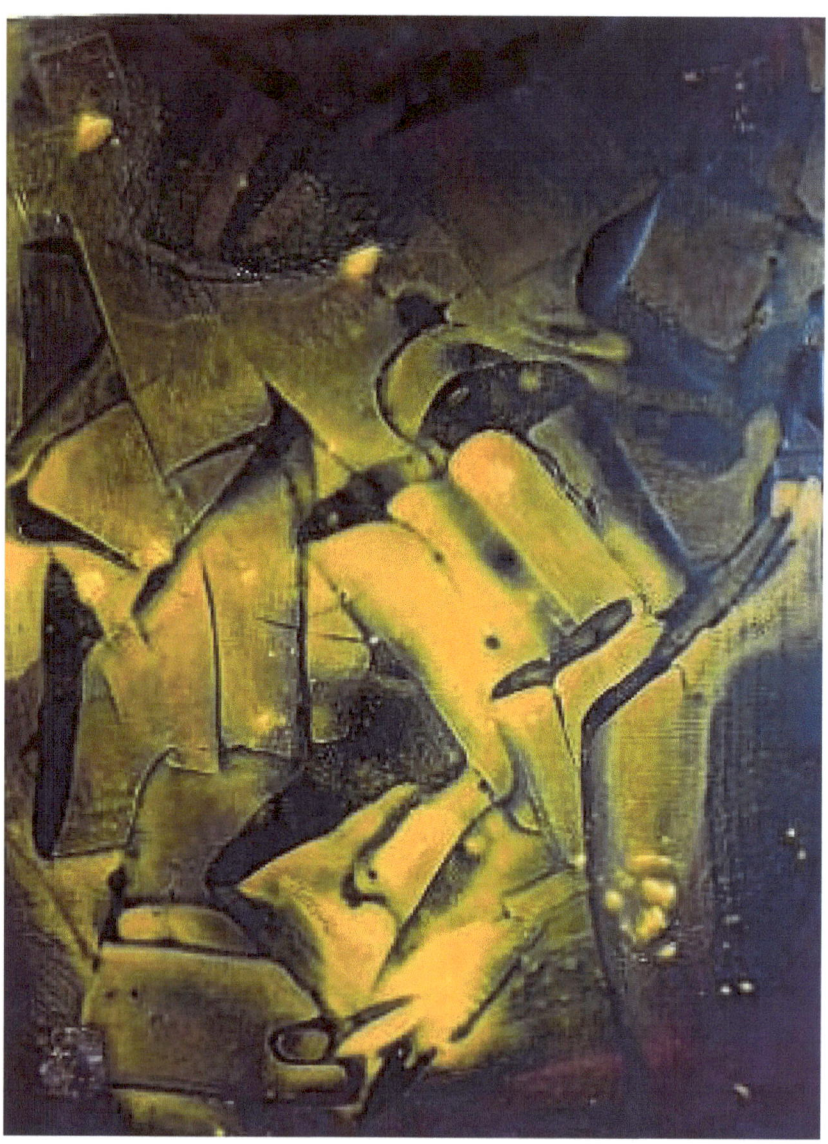

Nerve

A cordlike structure comprising a collection of nerve fibers that convey impulses between a part of the central nervous system and some other body regionl i.r. cranial roots from the side of the medulla oblongata, and by spinal roots from the side of the spinal cord (from the upper three or more cervical segments); the roots unite to form the trunk of the accessory nerve, which divides into an internal branch (cranial portion) and an external branch (spinal portion).

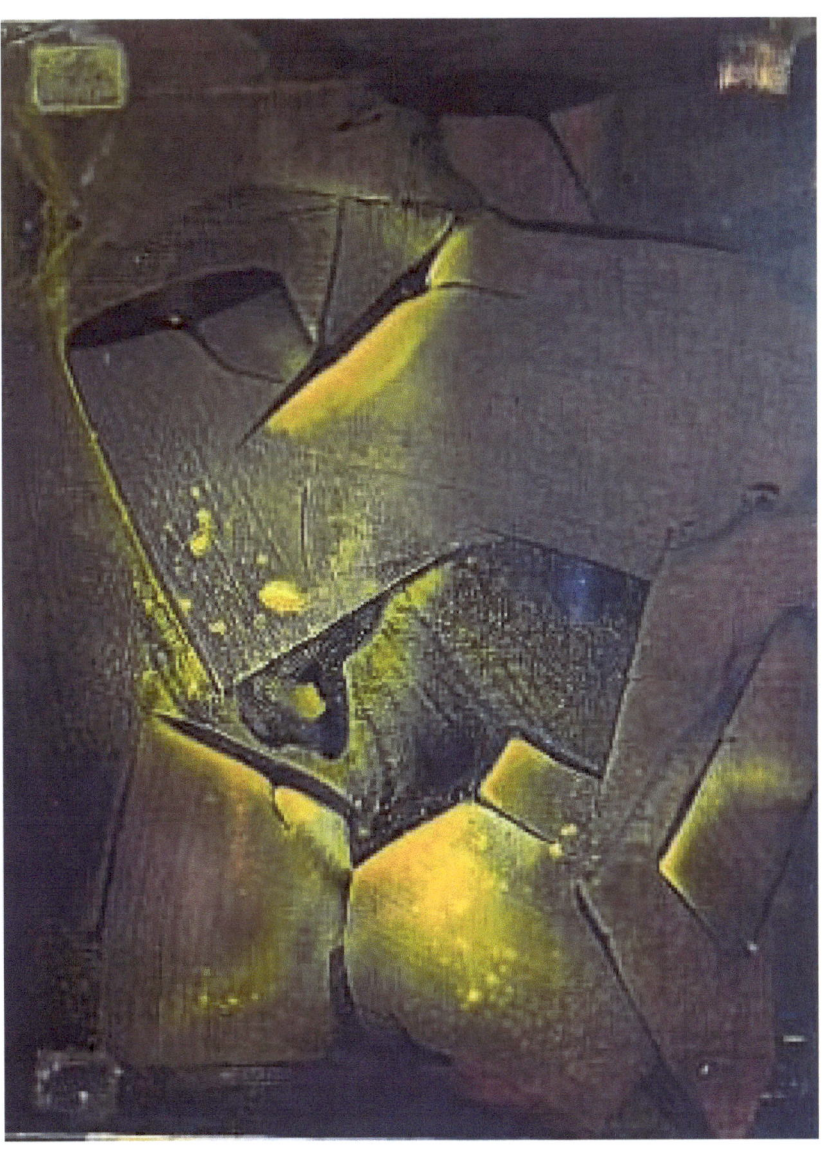

Ovary

One of the paired female gonads found on each side of the lower abdomen, beside the uterus in a fold of the broad ligament. At ovulation, an egg is expelled from a follicle on the surface of the ovary under the stimulation of the gonadotrophic hormones follicle-stimulating hormone (FSH) and luteinizing hormone (LH).

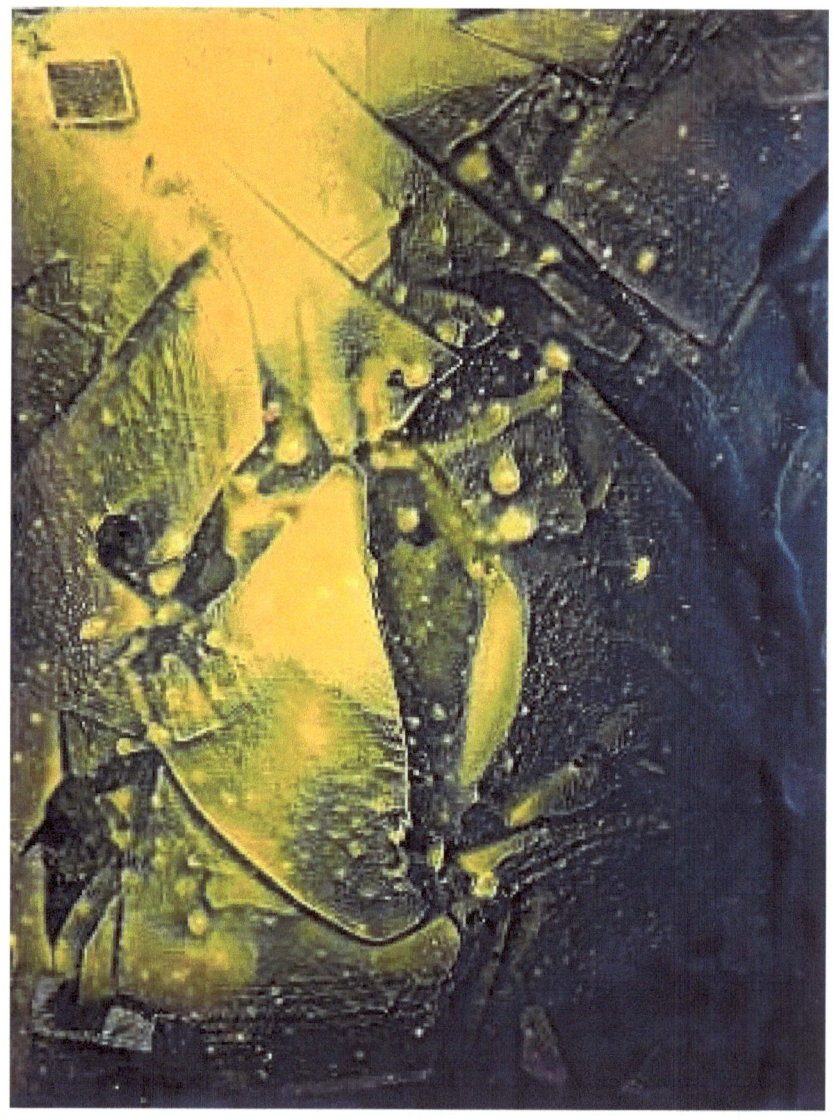

Pancreas

A large, elongated gland lying transversely behind the stomach, between the spleen and duodenum. Its external secretion contains digestive enzymes.

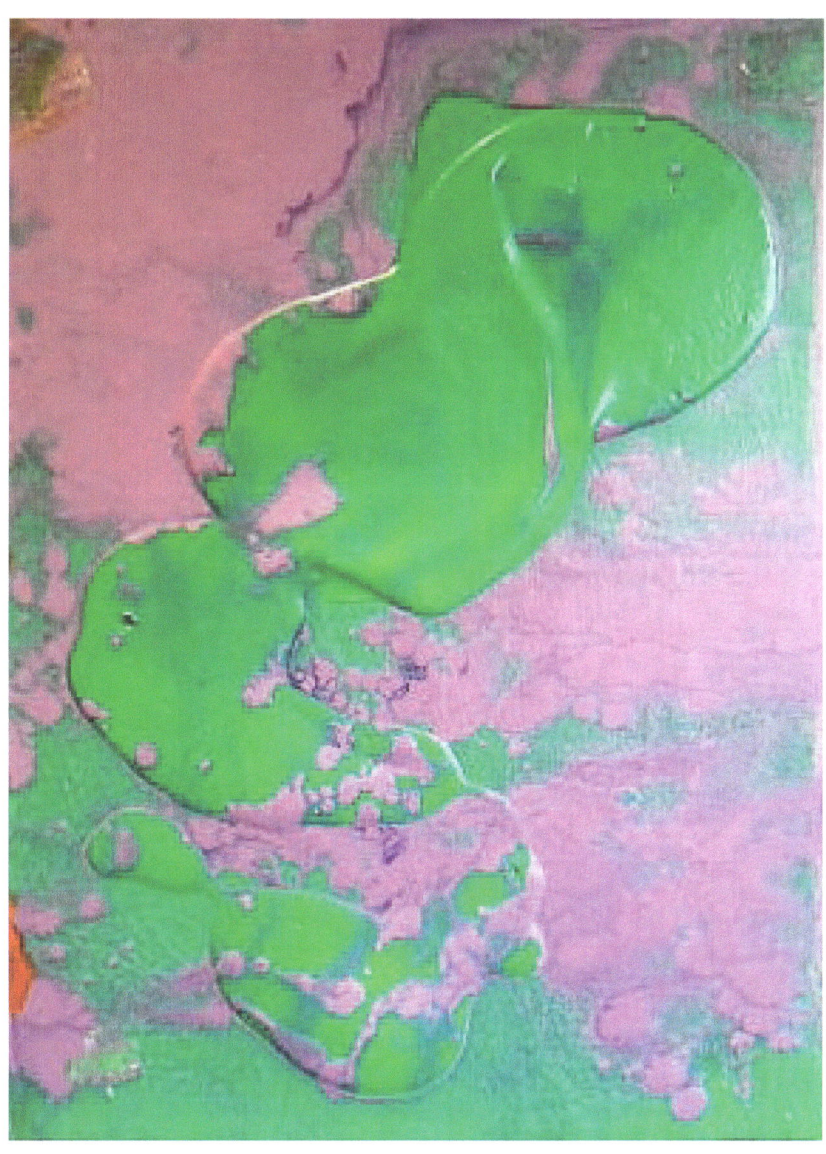

Phosphate

An organic compound necessary for mineralization of bone and other key cellular processes.

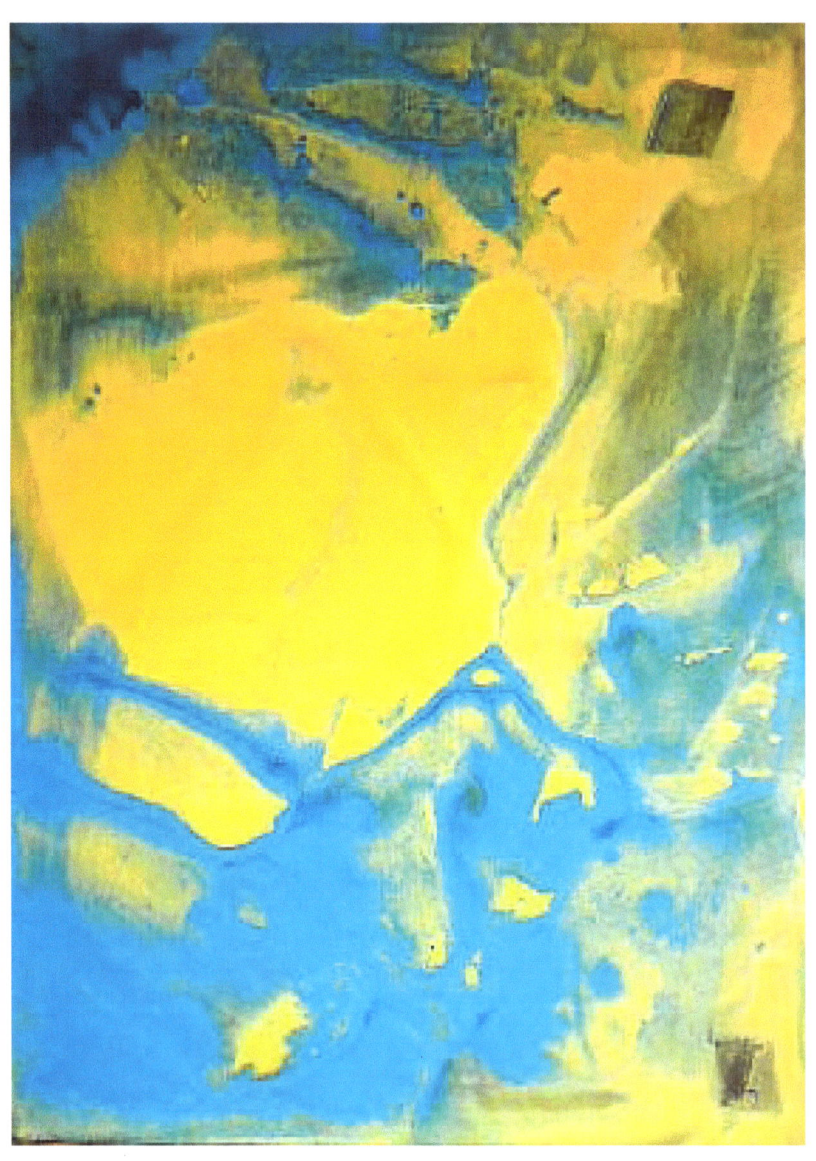

Plasma

Plasma makes up 50% of human blood. It is a watery fluid that carries red cells, white cells, and platelets throughout the body.

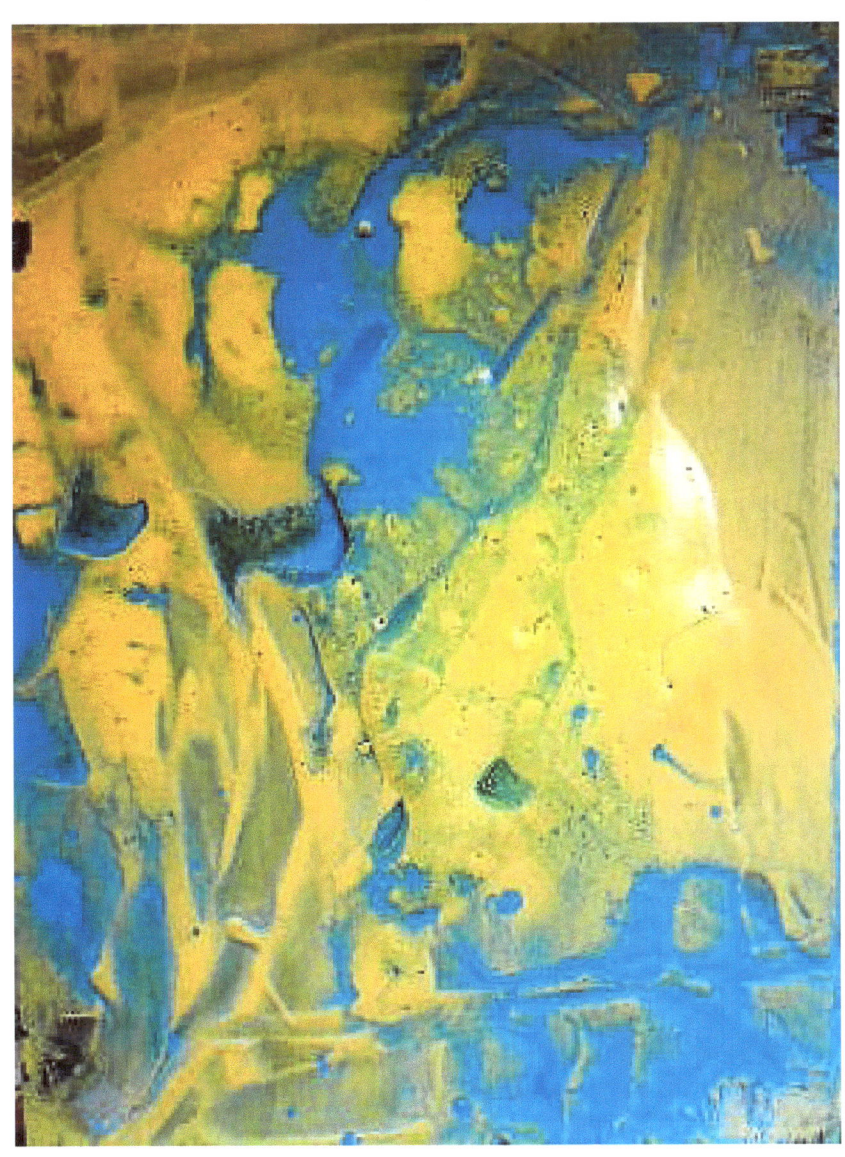

Prostate

A gland in men that surrounds the neck of the bladder and the proximal part of the urethra and produces a fluid that becomes part of semen. A firm structure normally about the size of a chestnut, the prostate is located in the pelvic cavity,

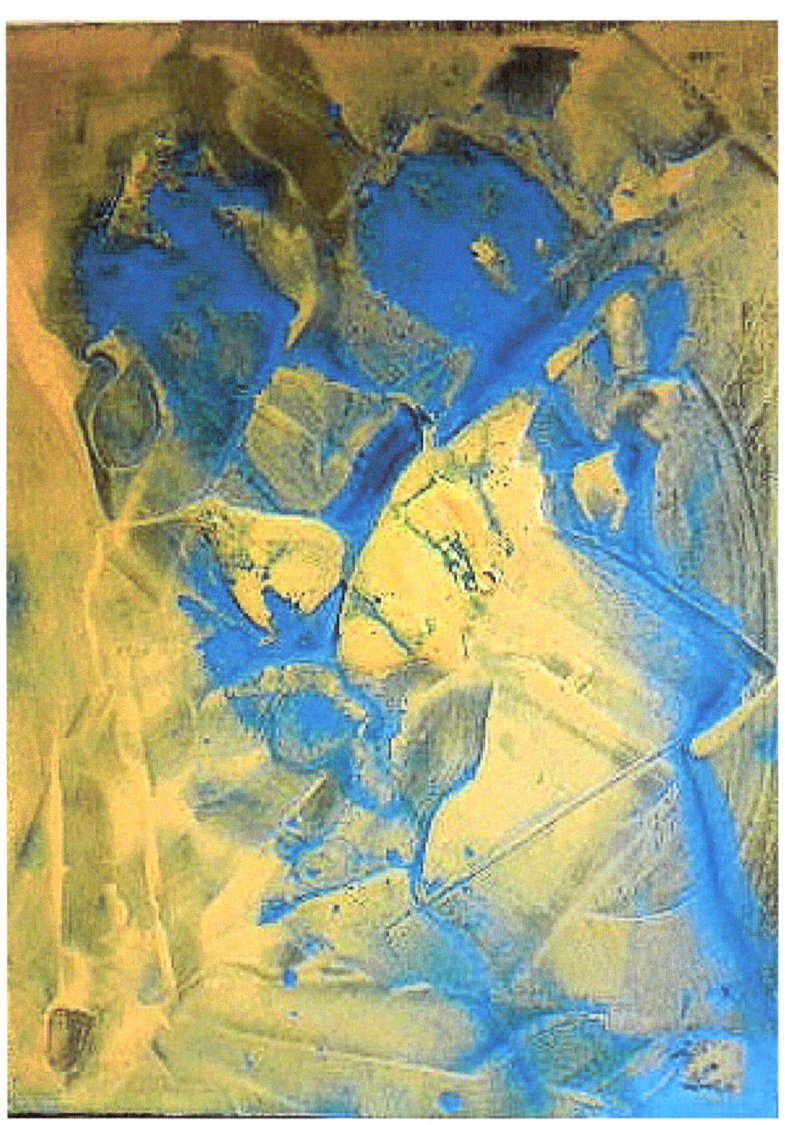

Receptors

A molecule on the surface or within a cell that recognizes and binds with specific molecules, producing a specific effect in the cell; e.g., the cell-surface receptors for antigens or cytoplasmic receptors for steroid hormones. A sensory nerve ending that responds to various stimuli.

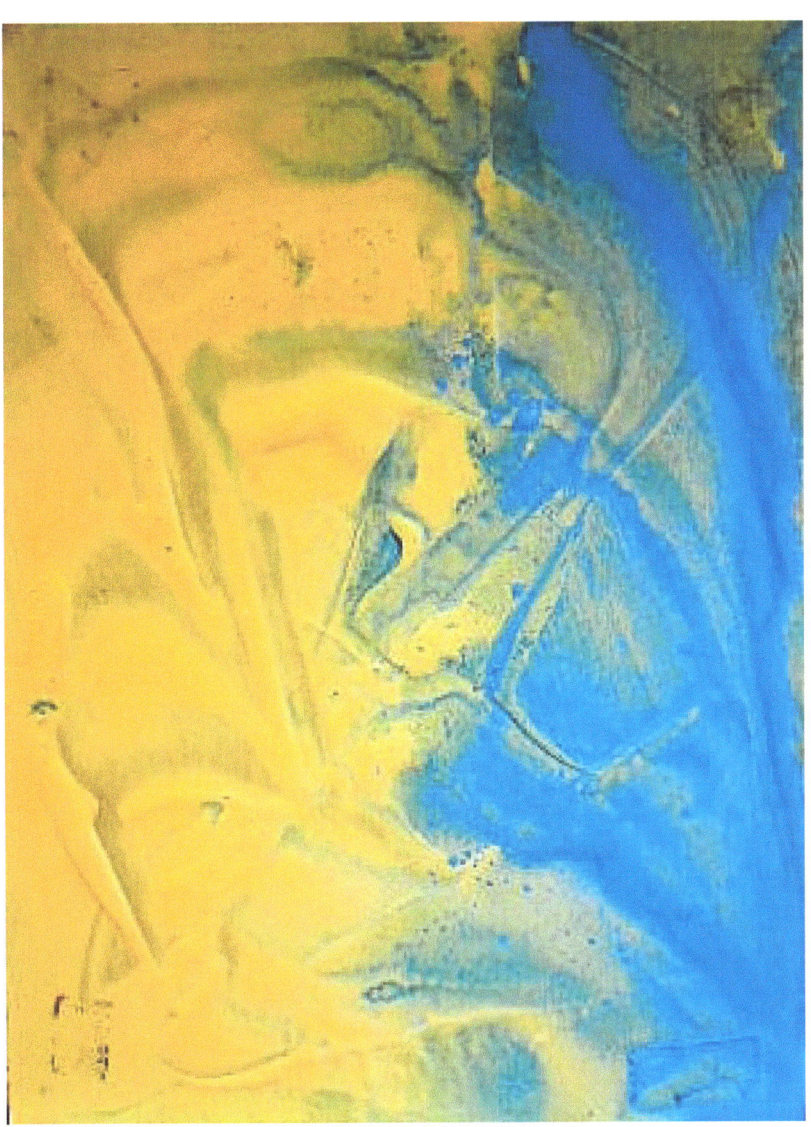

Saliva

The watery mixture of secretions from the salivary and oral mucous glands that lubricates chewed food, moistens the oral walls, and contains piyalin.

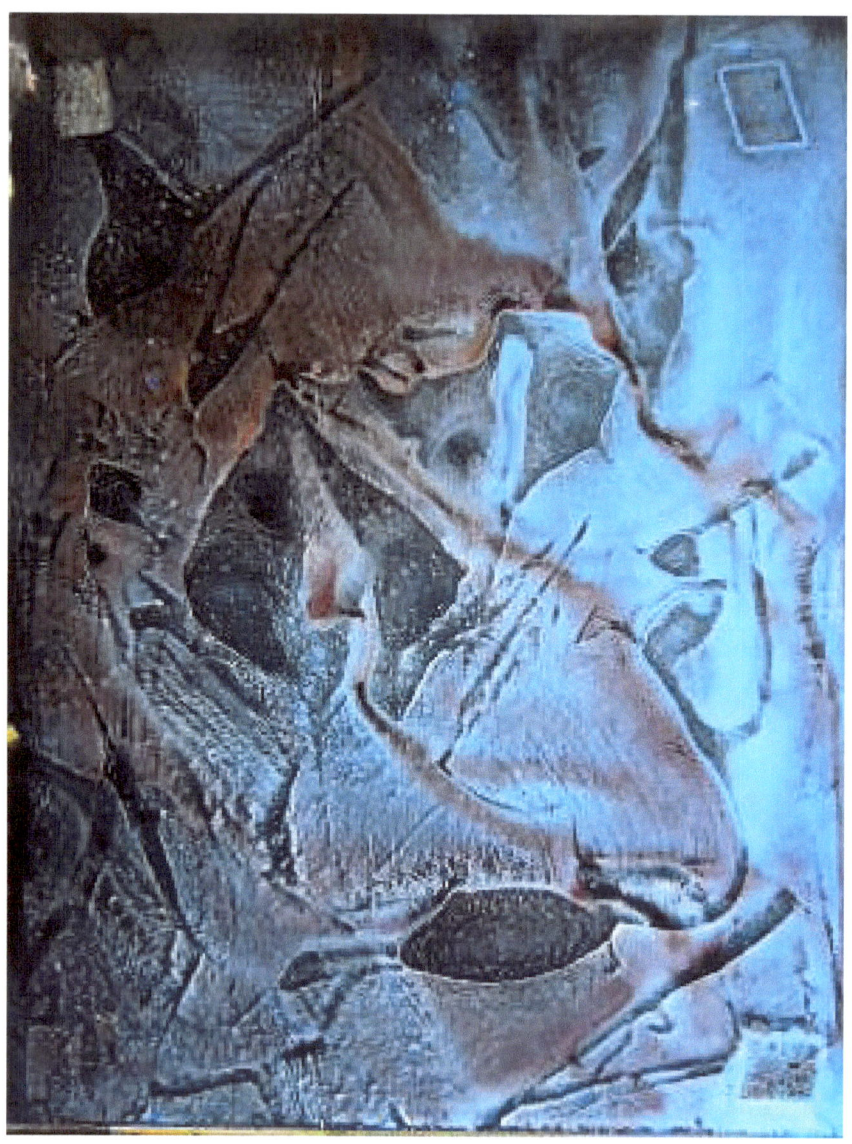

Semen

The thick, whitish secretion of the male reproductive organs discharged from the urethra during ejaculation. It contains spermatozoa in their nutrient plasma as well as secretions of the prostate, seminal vesicles, and other glands.

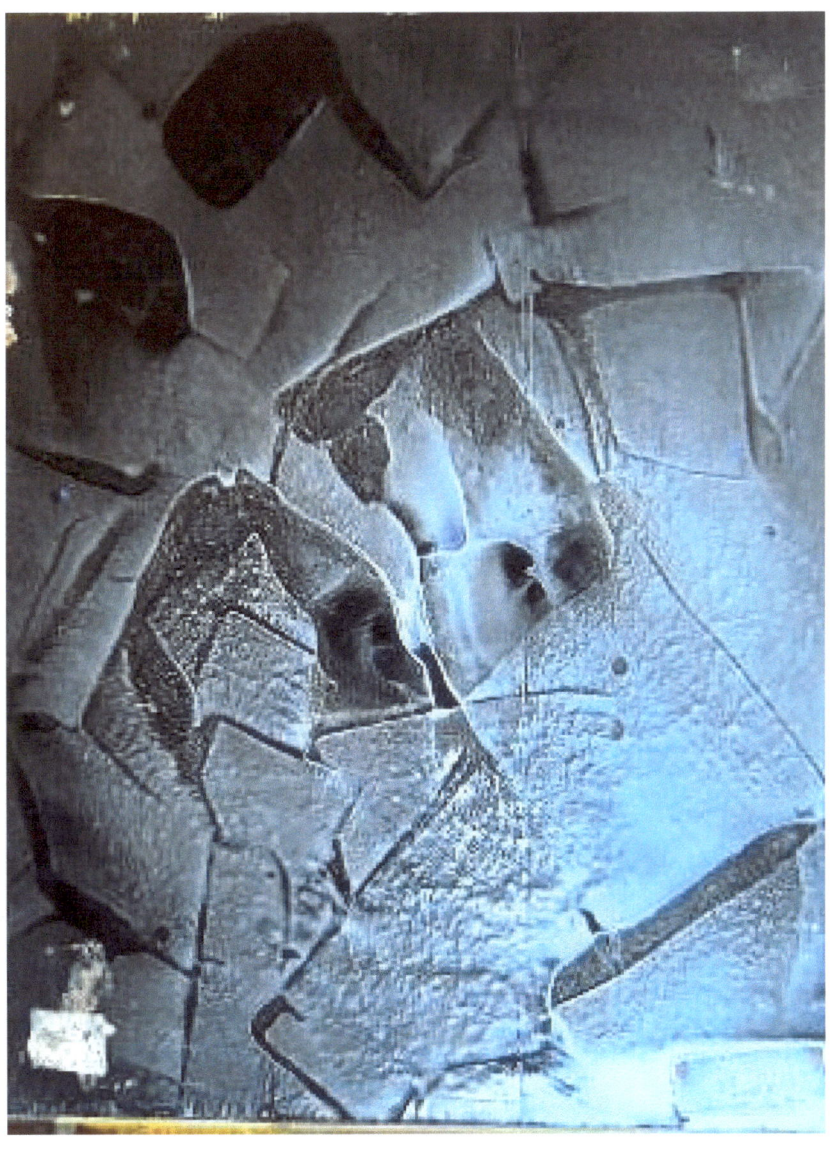

Synapse

The site of functional apposition between neurons, where an impulse is transmitted from one to another, usually by a chemical neurotransmitter released by the axon terminal of the presynaptic neuron.

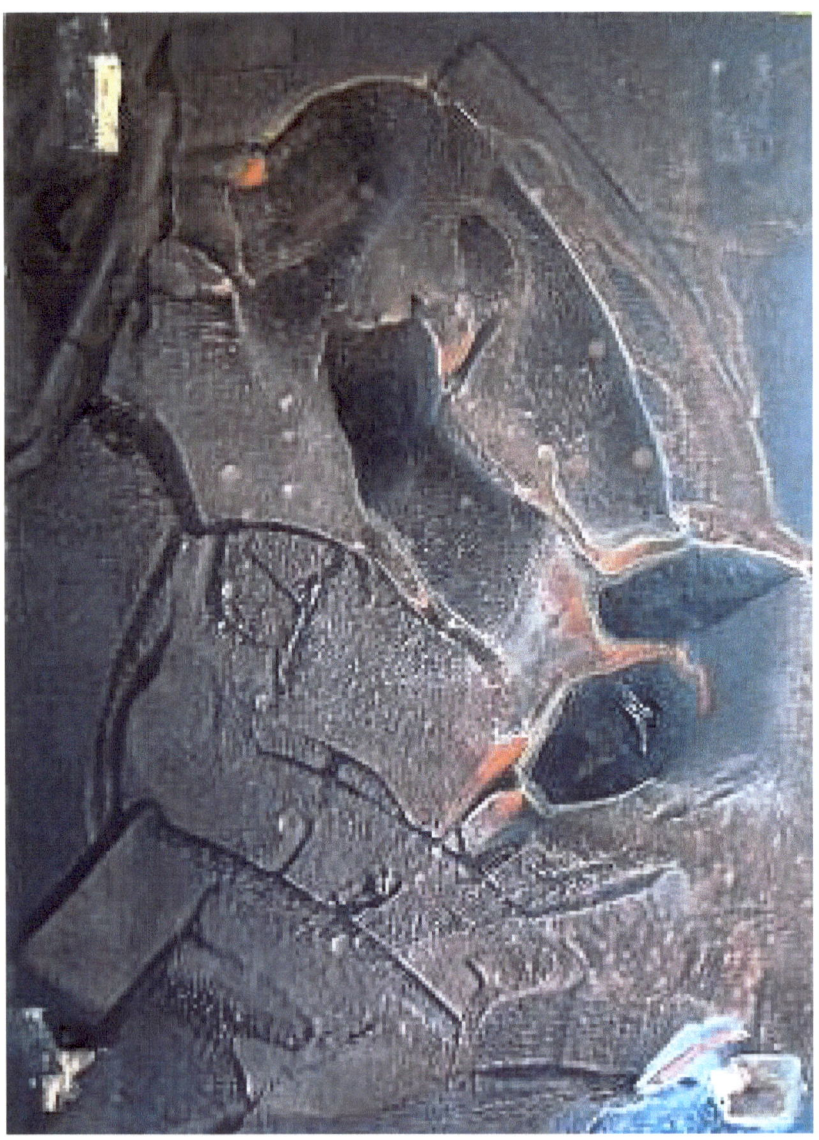

Sesamoid
A small nodular bone embedded in a tendon or joint capsule.

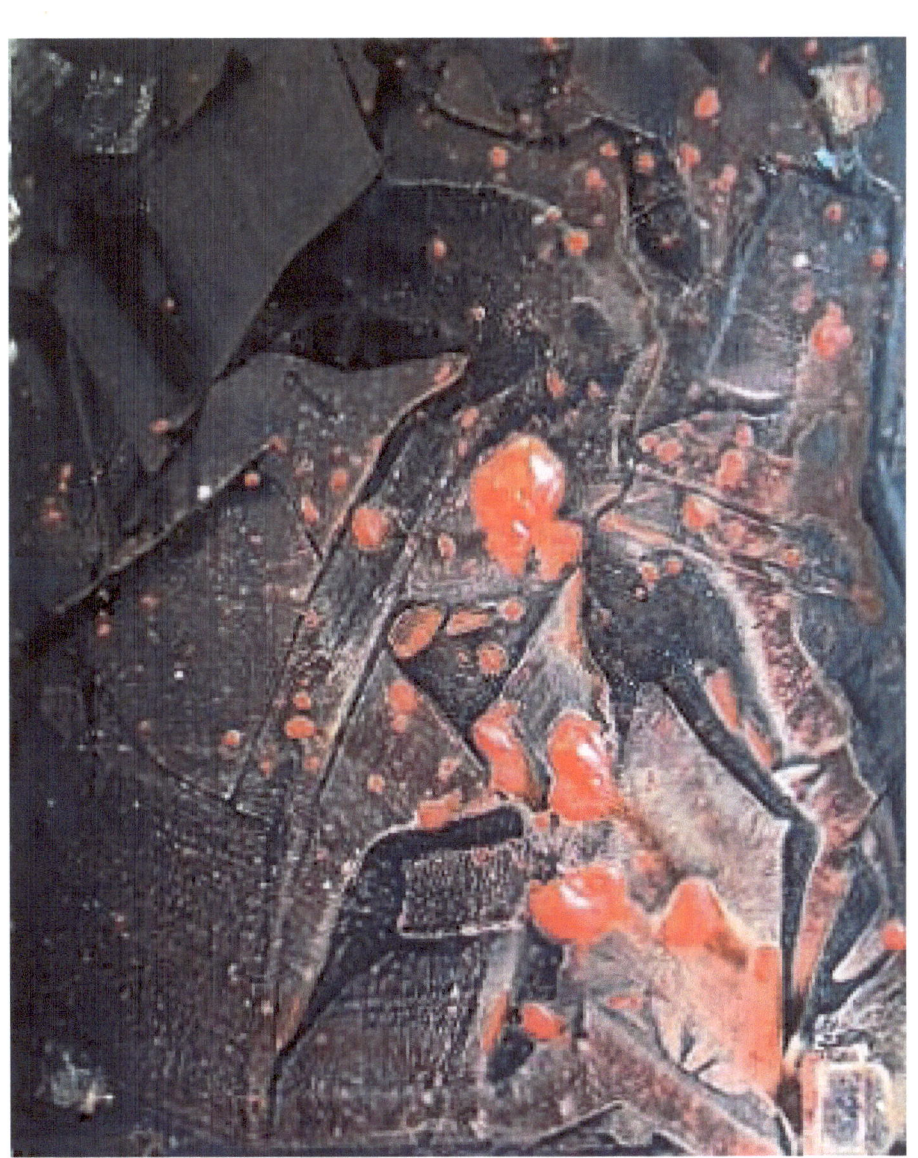

Spleen

A large, glandlike organ situated in the upper left part of the abdominal cavity, lateral to the cardiac end of the stomach. Among its functions are the disintegration of erythrocytes and the setting free of haemoglobin, which the liver converts into bilirubin; the genesis of new erythrocytes during fetal life and in the newborn; serving as a blood reservoir.

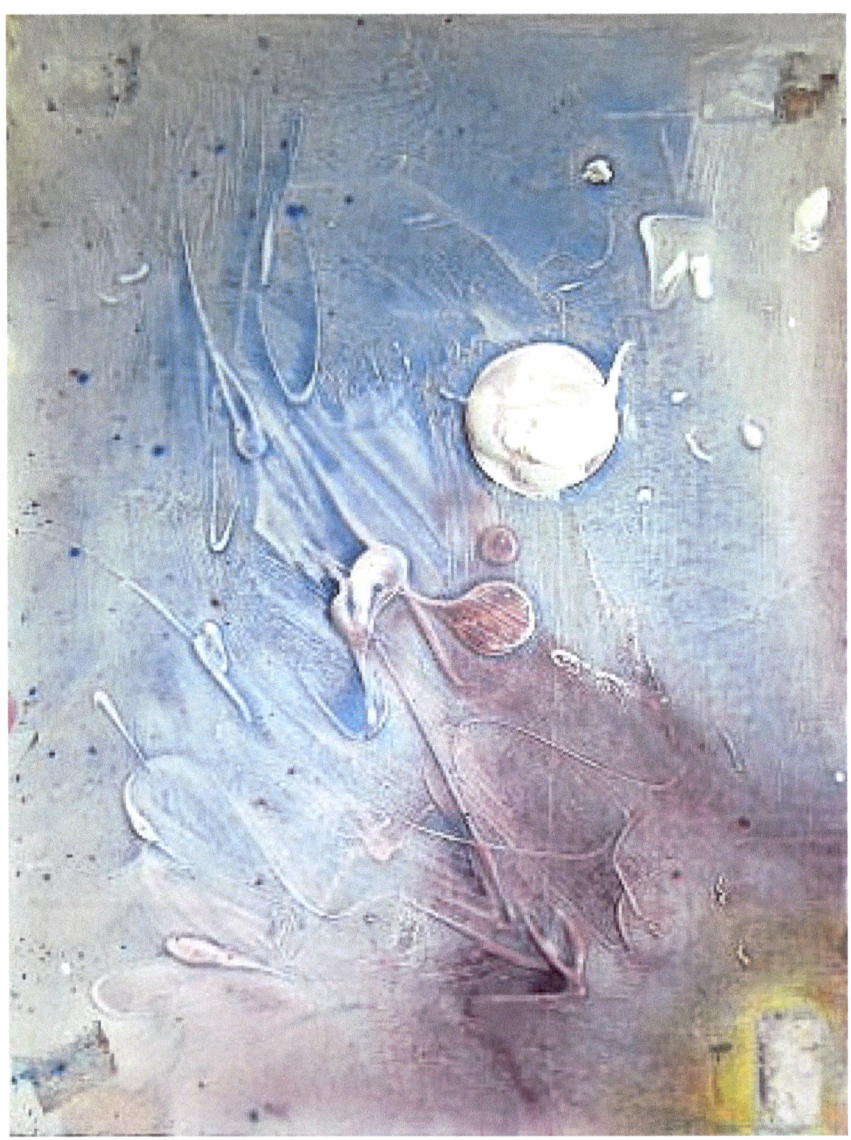

Sternum

A long flat bone, articulating with the cartilages of the first seven ribs and with the clavicle, forming the middle part of the anterior wall of the thorax, and consisting of the corpus, manubrium, and xiphoid process.

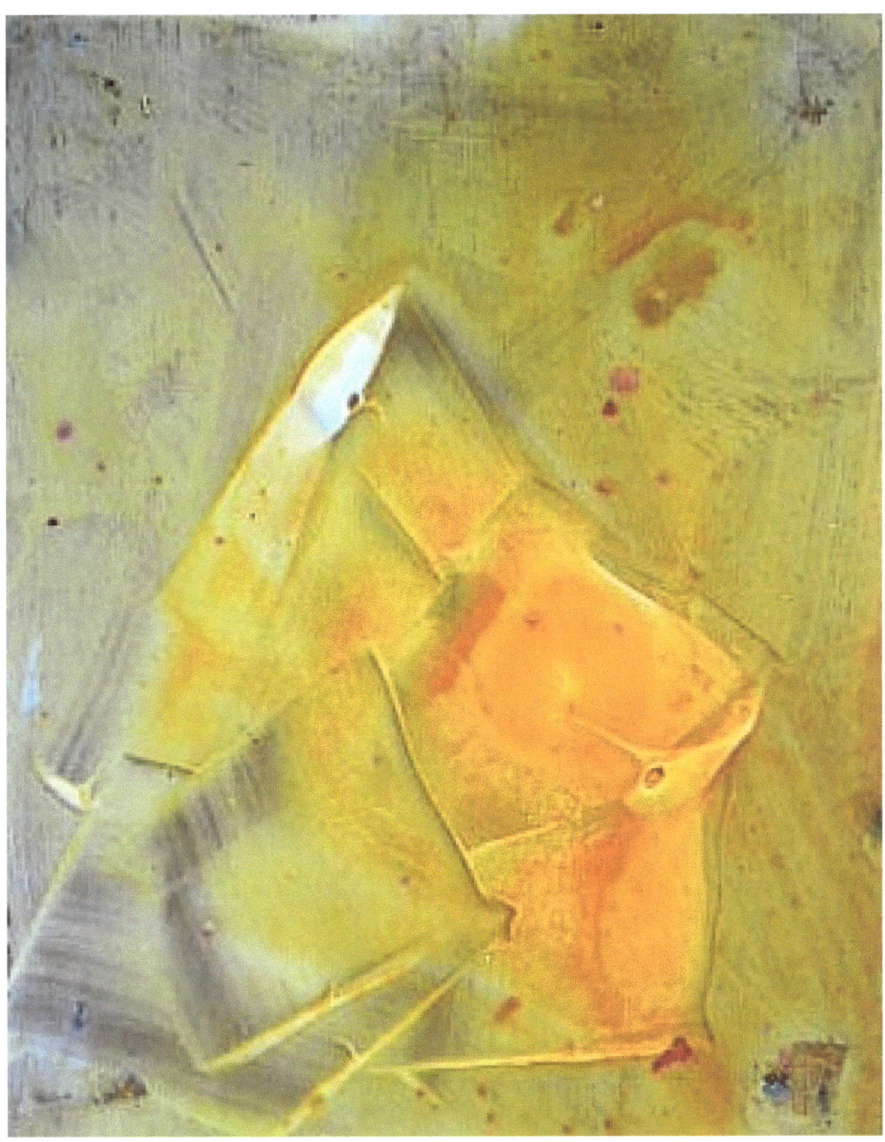

Taste Buds

any one of many peripheral taste organs distributed over the tongue, epiglottis, and the roof of the mouth. The five basic taste sensations registered by chemical stimulation of the taste buds are sweet, sour, bitter, savory, and salty.

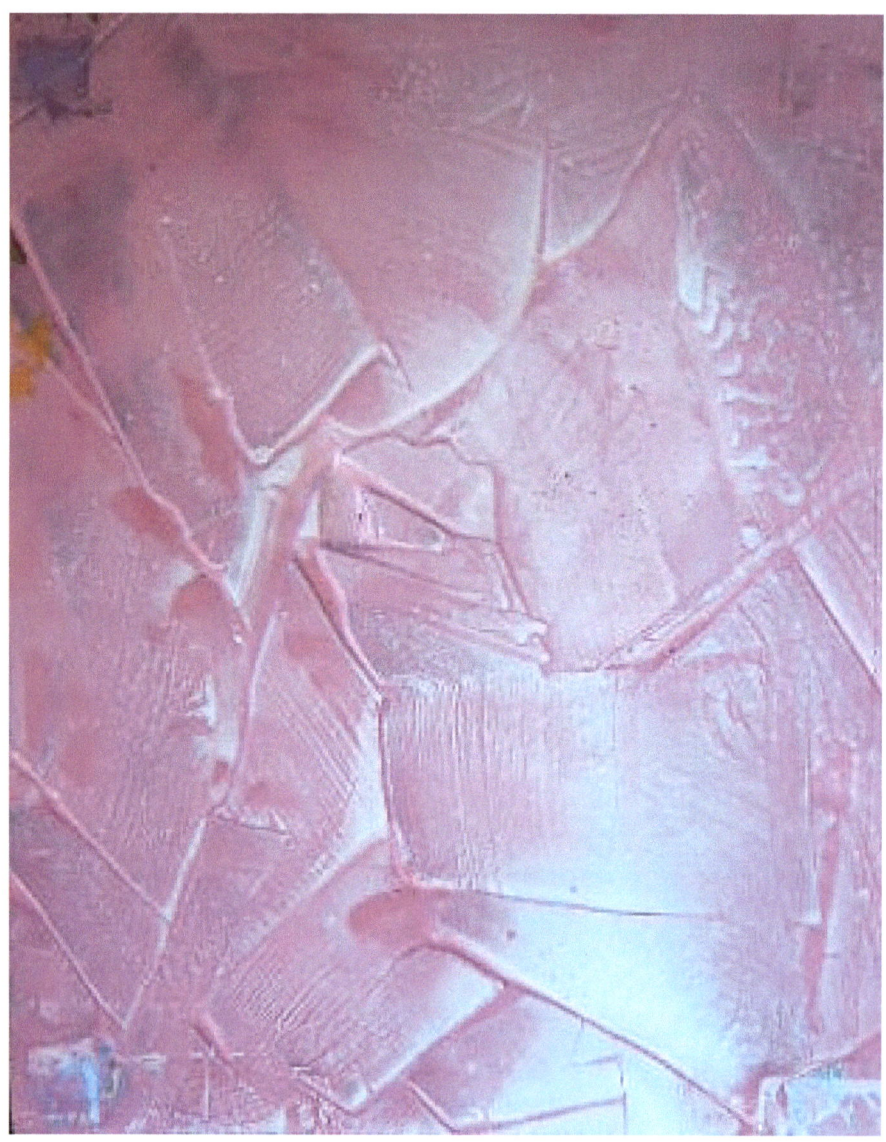

Testes
The male gonad; either of the paired egg-shaped glands normally situated in the scrotum, in which the spermatozoa develop.

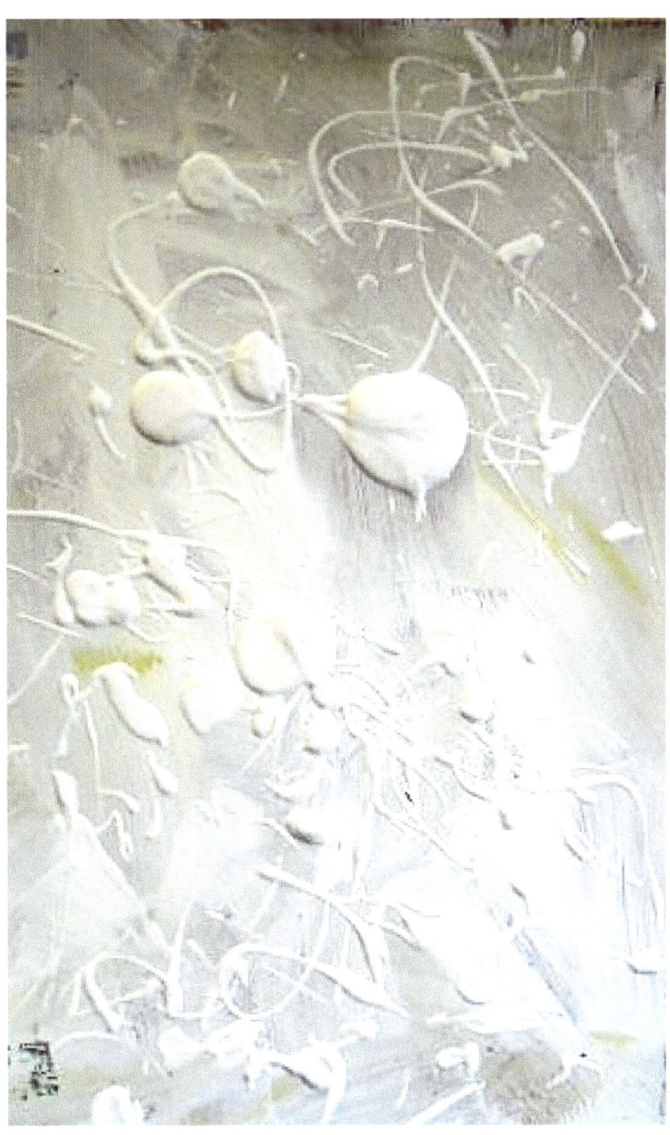

Tubules
Tissues and cells associated with the structures that connect the renal pelvis to the glomeruli.

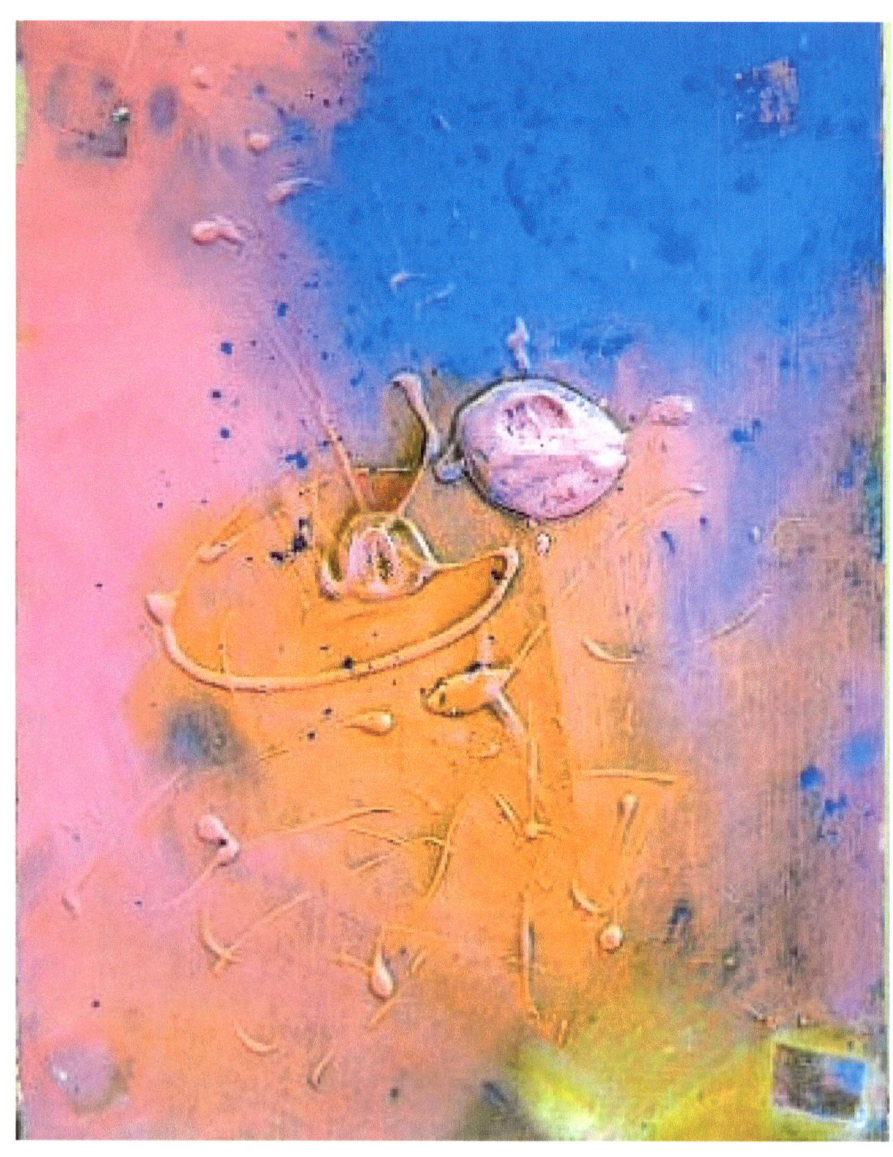

Urethra

The duct through which urine passes from the bladder to the outside of the body in most mammals and some fish and birds. In males, the urethra passes through the penis and also serves as the duct for the release of sperm, which enter the urethra from the vas deferens.

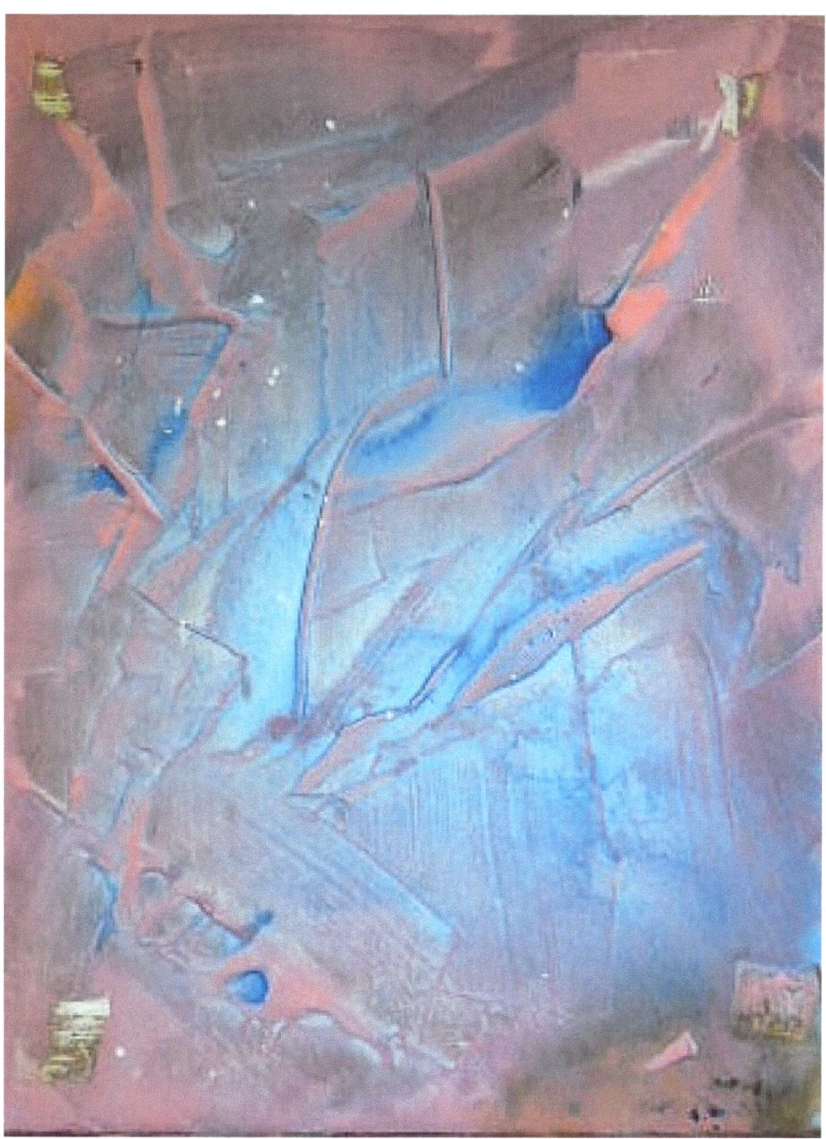

Uterus

The hollow muscular organ in female mammals in which the blastocyst normally becomes embedded and in which the developing embryo and fetus is nourished. Its cavity opens into the vagina below and into a uterine tube on either side.

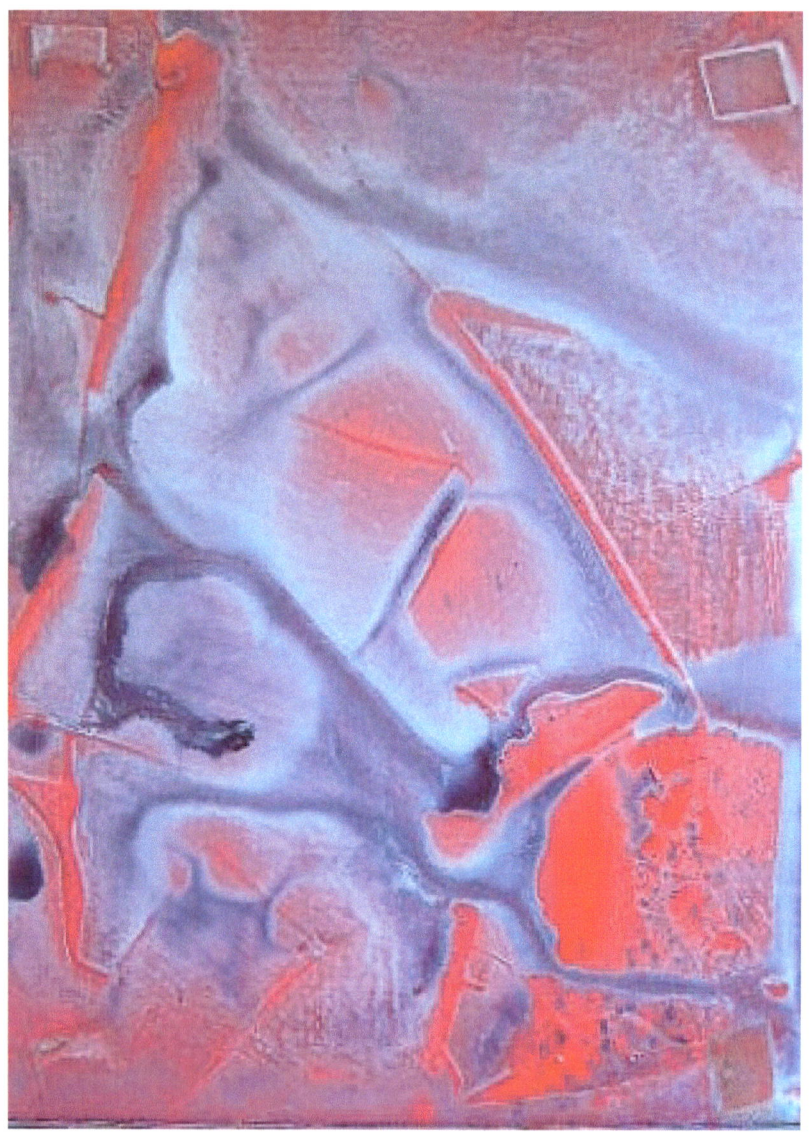

Vertebrae

Bones in the cervical, thoracic, and lumbar regions of the body that make up the vertebral column. Vertebrae have a central foramen (hole), and their superposition makes up the vertebral canal that encloses the spinal cord.

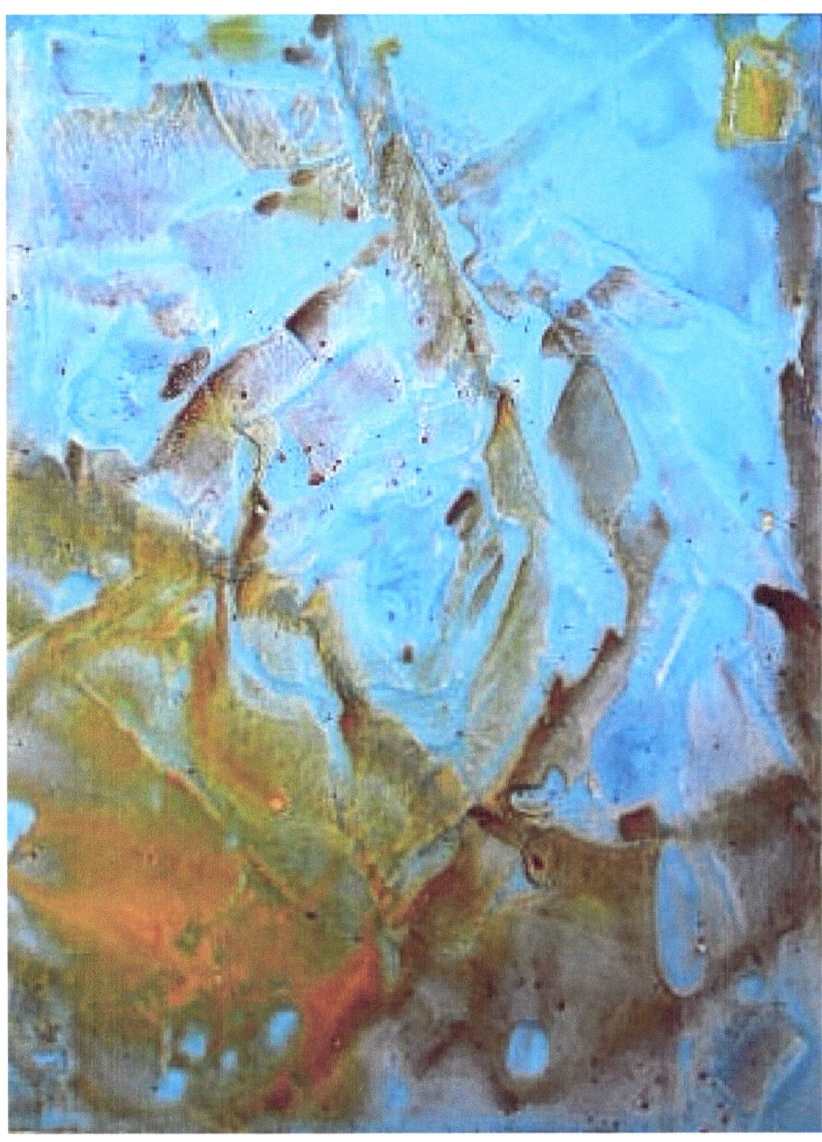

Womb

The upper part of the uterus is broad and flattened; the middle part (body), is large and open; and the lower part is narrow and tubular and opens downward into the Vagina. Two Fallopian Tubes enter the uterus at the upper end, one on each side. The walls of the uterus are composed of muscle, and its lining is mucous membrane. The muscular substance of the uterus is called the Myometrium and the inner lining is called the Endometrium.

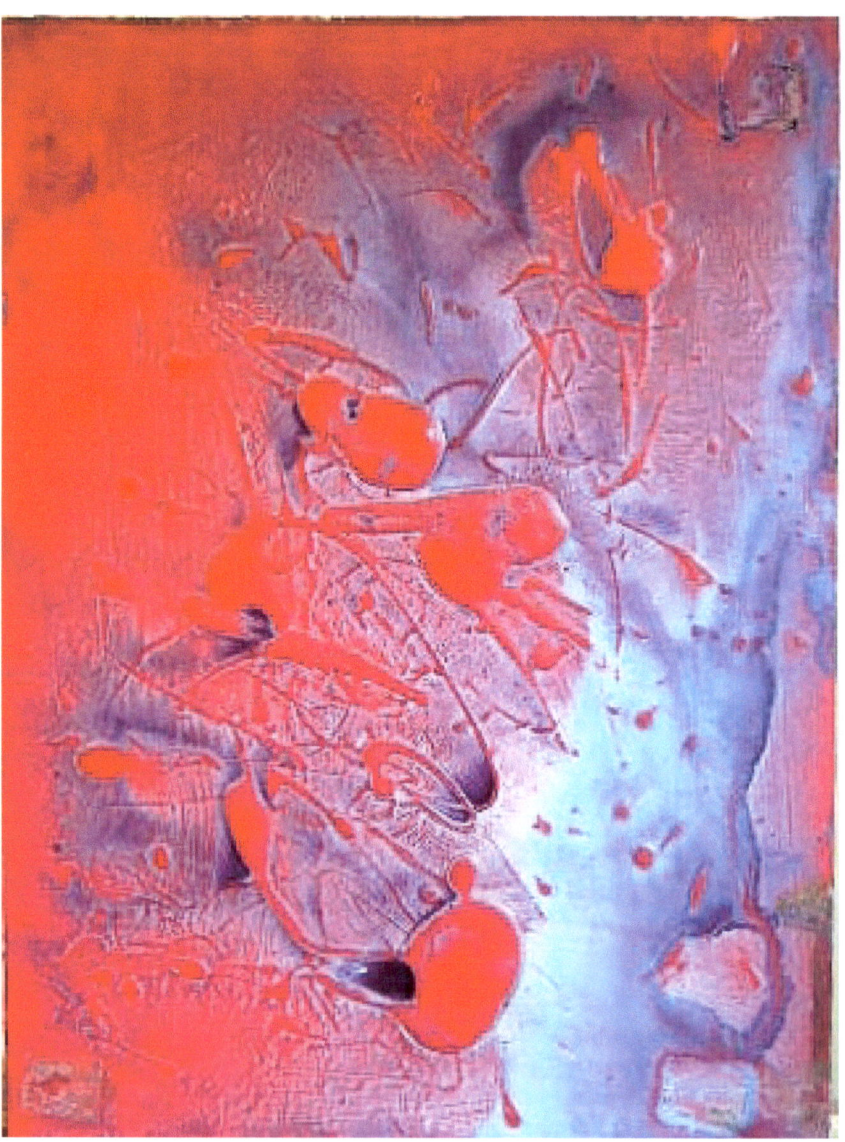

Artist Profile

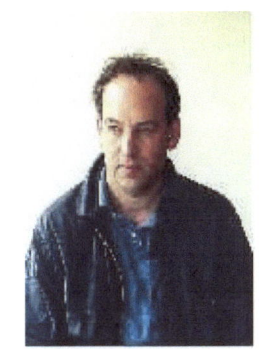

Born November1948, Bromley Kent Nicholas Philip James studied painting with Frank Auerbach and Keith Vaughan at the Slade School, UCL (BA), printmaking with Stanley Jones at the Curwen Press, and History of Art (MA) at Kingston University. His primary attraction to landscape developed in works made in the 1960s on site in Sussex, Devon, Cornwall and the Lake District progressing to city views of London and Paris. **1978-85** Assignments included 'Marine' themed paintings for the Bristol Bar chain USA (Gilbert Robinson Inc), *Boardroom Portrait* (Inchcape Plc), **1981** *The Guinness Portrait* (Arthur Guinness & Co 200th Anniversary) and continuing commissions. He regularly exhibits at The Royal Institute of Oil Painters (Winsor & Newton Prize 2003, elected a full member ROI 2006).

He has exhibited at The Wold Galleries, Gloucestershire, Courcoux and Courcoux, Stockbridge, The Turner Gallery, Exeter, and Whittington Fine Art Henley. In April 2008 with his sister Liz Summers at Peter Pears Gallery Aldeburgh, Suffolk,.Exhibitions in **2013** include Threadneedle Bank HQ *January-March and Royal Automobile Club Pall Mall and Woodcote Park February/December. The artist's prints are included in the Tate Britain archive (Curwen Gift) with publications on deposit with The British Library's media and book collections. His work is held in numerous private collections here and abroad. Entries include Dartmoor Artists (Brian Le Messurier, Hallsgrove Press) and Who's Who In Art (Hilmarton Manor Press).

Gallery Contact: The Federation of British Artists,
17 Carlton House Terrace, London SW1 020 7930 6844

Studio site: www.tracksdirectory.ision.co.uk/philipjames

Selected bibliographic sources with acknowledgements :
Moore Dalley: *Clinically Oriented Anatomy* (Lippincott,Wilkins & Willis)
Tyldesly & Grieve: *Muscles, Nerves & Movement* (Blackwell's Science)
Szunyoght/Feler *Human Anatomy For Artists* (Konemann)
Logan Dixon: *Human Sectional Anatomy* (OUP)
Sinnatanby: *Last's Anatomy* (Churchill Livingstone)
Alcamo: *Anatomy Coloring Workbook* (The Princeton Review)
The Free Dictionary www.thefreedictionary.com/

Other titles from Cv/Visual Arts Research

ART . TRAVEL . CAREERS . HISTORIES .
SOCIAL STUDIES . STUDIO WORK
Published by Cv Publications
Www.tracksdirectory.ision.co.uk

www.ingramcontent.com/pod-product-compliance
Lightning Source LLC
Chambersburg PA
CBHW051156220526
45473CB00003B/793